MIGRAINE HEADACHES
AND THE FOODS YOU EAT

200 Recipes for Relief

Agnes Peg Hartnell, EdD, RD, and G. Scott Tyler, MD

C H R O N I M E D   P U B L I S H I N G

Migraine Headaches and the Foods You Eat: 200 Recipes for Relief
© 1997 by Agnes Peg Hartnell and G. Scott Tyler

Library of Congress Cataloging-in-Publication Data

Migraine headaches and the foods you eat/ Agnes Peg Hartnell, EdD, RD, and G. Scott Tyler, MD
        p.   cm.
Includes index.
ISBN 1-56561-121-7 $12.95

Edited by: Jolene Steffer and Jeff Braun
Cover Design: Pear Graphics
Text Design & Production: David Enyeart
Art/Production Manager: Claire Lewis
Printed in the United States of America

Published by
Chronimed Publishing
P.O. Box 59032
Minneapolis, MN 55459-0032

Notice: Consult a Health Care Professional

Because individual cases and needs vary, readers are advised to seek the guidance of a licensed physician, registered dietitian, or other health care professional before making changes in their health care regimens. This book is intended for informational purposes only and is not for use as an alternative to appropriate medical care. While every effort has been made to ensure that the information is the most current available, new research findings, being released with increasing frequency, may invalidate some data.

For all their special help, and love—the Verlin P. Jenkins family,
Hanna Hartnell, Jan, Brian, and Shannon Hancock

Acknowledgments

Much gratitude is due to the dietitians who gave us permission to see their original materials which we adapted for this book, especially Pam McCarthy, RD, and Ann Moore Allen, RD.

Current, varied periodical references and expert assistance were provided by Frances Reay, Cathy Corak Shumard, Karolyn Frye, Sue Zevan, Joanne Hagmann, Elaine Kvitka Nevins, Jan Hancock, Lee Fischer, Karin Wade, and Millie Krull.

Our thanks to the dedicated and professional staff at Chronimed Publishing, especially Cheryl Kimball, Jeff Braun, and Claire Lewis.

Table of Contents

Introduction

DO YOU HAVE frequent, severe headaches, including migraine? Do you know anyone else who does? Almost everybody seems to know someone with migraine headaches.

Each year headache sufferers spend about $400 million on over-the-counter medications. Studies indicate that half of the 45 million Americans who suffer headaches do not seek a physician's help. Nearly 90 percent could be treated successfully.

After treating headache patients for 30 years, Scott Tyler, M.D., became convinced that certain foods could trigger headaches. (Within the last few years, as Chapter 1 shows, many other physicians have reached the same conclusion.) So Dr. Tyler decided to collaborate with Dr. Agnes Peg Hartnell, a registered dietitian and home economist, and compile this headache prevention book.

In this book none of the twelve established headache-triggering foods is used in the recipes. Moreover, as an extra precaution, additional ingredients that have been found dangerous to some are marked with an asterisk in the recipes.

This headache control book, as far as we can determine, is the first and only book written for today's lifestyle with three types of recipes:

- ❑ Quick and Easy Recipes, some of which may take no longer to prepare than eat (some include microwave instructions)
- ❑ Prepare Ahead Recipes, which usually take a bit longer to prepare
- ❑ Specialty Recipes (Gourmet/Creative)

While most people value these recipes for the freedom they offer from headache-triggering ingredients, their lack of commercial additives, emulsifiers, preservatives, etc., makes the foods nutritionally superior to "fast" foods, either purchased or prepared. And because these recipes feature natural foods and are free of additives, they can be of great benefit to all members of the family, not only those who suffer from headaches.

Furthermore, knowing that food costs are always on the rise, the recipes and menus are economical in most cases.

Migraine Versus Other Headaches

In this book we don't necessarily differentiate between migraine and other types of headaches. After all, there possibly is no difference in the cause of the migraine and other types of headaches such as cluster and muscle contraction or tension headaches: dietary management applies to them all!

There is one theory, however, that migraine "washes" from decreased blood flow (spreading electrical depression) from a small region at the rear of the brain. Further research is required, but it is interesting to note that in animal studies, one of the three stimuli was amino acids (protein particles) as found naturally in certain foods.

For all people with migraines, exercising daily, eating breakfast, getting sufficient sleep, and other healthy wellness habits may be as good as medicine in reducing the frequency and severity of migraine headaches. What about the recently approved migraine cure, sumatriptan, and others awaiting government acceptance? It is our experience that most people prefer prevention to cures, especially with new medications that have not stood the test of time and may have potentially harmful side-effects. Even so, consult your doctor for diagnosis and treatment options.

If your physician is not familiar with the principles underlying the program, you may wish to show him or her this book so you can work together using these concepts. Chapters 1 and 2 explain how food ingredients cause headaches. Chapter 3 adds information about medications and other non-food substances that can bring on headaches. Chapter 4 lists the foods to avoid, and the rest of the book gives more than 200 recipes that are designed to fit into your total program for headache prevention. Choose one of the recipes and start today. Bon appetit!

PART ONE

Migraine Prevention

Getting It Right, Getting It Done!

CHAPTER ONE

Is Your Diet Causing Your Headaches?

FORTUNATELY, THERE HAS BEEN an explosion in the amount of knowledge about the role of nutrition and health, including headaches, in the past decade. But why is the relationship between headaches and diet not yet universally recognized? As with any newer information, how can a person judge whether it's fact or fiction?

One test of the validity of a health claim is to check the scientific studies that back up the claim. Therefore, it is important to know the reputations of the scientist(s) who conducted the study and whether the study is published in a reputable scientific journal. These journals do not publish a study unless it has been reviewed and passed by other researchers.

Medical breakthroughs are broadcast and published in both the scientific and popular media and press. The remainder of this chapter reports reputable studies regarding the connection between headaches and nutrition from both types of publications. Their sources are also given so you can read the original reports.

Investigating Migraines and their Causes

According to *Taber's Medical Dictionary*, migraine is defined as an attack of headache usually accompanied by disordered vision and gastrointestinal upset… and may be the result of dilation of the cranial (brain) arteries… and may be precipitated by allergic hypersensitivity or emotional disturbances.

This 1985 definition is broader than many previous references that found no relationship between headaches and allergic hypersensitivity. Emotional or physical disturbances, causing stress, had been widely accepted as a cause of headache; most practitioners now accept that heredity is also an important factor.

Still, "headaches can be triggered by what you eat," says John Brainard, M.D., in the 1979 book, *Control of Migraine*. Five years later, another medical doctor, William J. Stump, contributed to a headache cookbook in which the main emphasis was on diet and the role food played in causing headaches.

Neil Solomon, M.D., a former *Los Angeles Times* health columnist, advised in 1990 that headaches might be helped by diagnosis and treatment involving food, chemical, mold, and yeast allergies for hypersensitivities. In one of his columns, Dr. Solomon pointed out the individuality of headache sufferers: men and women respond differently to the same drug (or food) so "it is possible a different medication or diet would be prescribed for each." Airplane food, in particular, earned Dr. Solomon's caution: "If you are subject to food-induced headache attacks, it would also be a good idea for you to bring along some food of your own on air travel trips. The in-flight food ordinarily contains a number of additives for flavor and these chemicals can precipitate a headache."

In 1988, *Environmental Nutrition*, a professional newsletter of diet, nutrition, and health, printed an article titled, "Can Migraines Be Managed Through Diet? Foods that May Be to Blame." It reported that while the exact causes of headaches remain unclear, a large number of experts believe that certain components of the diet may trigger headaches. "Food additives and some naturally-occurring substances in food could be the culprits.…"

Another medical practitioner, Loraine Stern, in the popular magazine *Women's Day*, wrote in the magazine's *Medical Facts Guide* that certain foods may contribute to migraines, most notably foods containing the chemical tyramine, which is present in many types of cheese, especially ripe cheese such as Camembert, Cheddar, and blue cheese.

Seymour Diamond, M.D., a headache specialist, has noted that in some persons low blood glucose levels can trigger a headache.

Registered dietitians, in addition to medical physicians, have written diet and meal plans to control headaches. Betty Wedman, R.D., says that one rule of thumb for headache sufferers is: the more simple and natural the food, the less likely it will contain chemicals or salt that could cause an allergic (histamine) response.

Carol A. Foster, M.D., of Valley Neurological Headache Clinic, listed a change in diet as one of the effective tools for treating headaches at an exhibit on a two-year national tour that started at the National Museum of Health and Medicine in Washington, D.C., with a kick off by former U.S. Surgeon General C. Everett Koop. In fact, "a person who suffers four to five headaches a month can see a 50-percent reduction in attacks by simply controlling his or her diet," says Frederick Freitag, M.D.

And finally, some words from Joel Saper, M.D., director of the Michigan Head Pain and Neurological Institute in Ann Arbor and author of the 1987 book, *Help for Headaches*: "Most headaches are due to disturbances in brain chemistry. That refines earlier views which blamed headaches on swelling of blood vessels or muscle tension. These changes can be involved, but they are triggered by quirks in the brain's messenger chemicals, according to the new view."

Dr. Saper points out that genetics make some people more susceptible than others. However, other factors such as medicine and food also play a role. He concludes that the new understanding of headaches is taking them out of the realm of psychological illness and putting them in the realm of a genetically determined (80 percent) biological illness.

In Dr. Saper's advice on headaches, he includes this question: "Look at past headaches and keep notes on future ones and see if there's a pattern as to when they occur... after eating certain foods or taking certain medicines? Drinking something with caffeine or alcohol? Cigarettes?" Certainly, there have been many different approaches to headaches through history. And no doubt there will be new recommendations in the years to come, but most specialists agree that diet and headaches have a strong connection. Hopefully this review will encourage you to try a new lifestyle, one that is free from the dietary triggers of headaches.

CHAPTER TWO

Why Some Foods Produce Migraines

SOME PEOPLE—often because of genetic inheritance—lack the ability or dietary enzymes to change some chemicals into harmless nutrients or chemicals in the body. These chemicals can be found in certain medications or naturally, in some foods.

These particular drugs or foods, if not counteracted by medications, can act as messengers and trigger headaches. They can be:

(1) irritating agents (similar to how pollen can cause hay fever), or

(2) blood vessel dilators (pressor agents) or blood pressure elevators

The head's bony skull cannot expand to accommodate the swelling of the circulatory system. The increased swelling in the skull is caused by either one or both of the triggers.

The brain itself isn't hurting, because it has no nerves for experiencing pain. However, the arteries in the brain do have pain nerves, and pain signals can be transferred to the conscious center of the brain with every heartbeat.

What are the chemicals in foods or medications that can produce headaches in sensitive individuals? One way that specifically irritating foods were discovered in the 1970s was through the use of an antidepressant medication called monoamine oxidase inhibitor (MAOI). This drug inhibits the action of an enzyme system in the liver that "digests" one of the brain's messenger chemicals, serotonin.

Normally, the liver changes the potentially harmful serotonin, found in some foods, into a harmless substance. "However, in the presence of this anti-depressant medication, MAOI, the body's defenses against serotonin are removed. If serotonin isn't neutralized by the body, its effect might be enhanced one hundred-fold. The patient develops a serious increase in blood pressure, headache, and even brain hemorrhage." The serotonin-sensitive individual can react the same, even without the MAOI inhibitor medication.

In addition to serotonin, other potent headache messengers have been found. These include protein particles (pressor agents) such as tyramine, tyrosine, dopamine, caffeine, glutamine, histamine, phenylethylamine, fermented foods, yeasts, and aged foods where protein breakdown occurs. Bacteria themselves, which are involved in the breakdown of protein, are capable of acting as headache trigger agents, too.

According to the book *Food-Medications Interactions*, the irritating content generally increases as a protein-rich food ages and may undergo protein degradation if stored too long or contaminated. Cooking of degraded protein does not destroy the irritant, so it is recommended that perishable refrigerated items be consumed within 48 hours of purchase.

Thus, in susceptible persons, diet-triggered headaches are linked to the defective use of certain protein particles (amines). The resulting toxic products can also be caused by other foods that contain protein particles (without the action of bacteria), such as a few fruits and vegetables. In addition, sodium (commonly found in salt) and nitrates and nitrites (in smoked foods) are common headache triggers for some people.

Interestingly, some irritating foods contain weak triggering chemicals, often in small quantities. These foods are unlikely to cause problems unless eaten in large amounts. Many people find they can tolerate a small amount, approximately 1/2 cup (4 ounces) or less, of the offending food and no more frequently than once a week. However, there is no guarantee that the same foods will not produce a severe reaction in the future.

The offending chemical content also can vary from product to product of the same class and even between samples of the same product. For example, the portions of cheese closer to the rind have a much higher tyramine content than those further from the rind. Dairy products such as sour cream and yogurt may or may not be irritating, depending upon their age and process of manufacture.

To add to the confusion in discovering which particular foods a person is sensitive to, stress is a factor. Stress of any kind, especially emotional or physical, varies enough to lower the threshold for a migraine attack one time and not for another time with the same food.

So what are the foods that contain the agents or chemicals that may have a connection to migraine? The lists can be divided into three categories:

1. Foods to be Avoided by Most
2. Foods to be Consumed with Caution
3. Foods Dangerous to Some

As you read this list of foods that must be avoided, you'll naturally wonder what you *can* eat. Thankfully, there is a longer list of "allowed foods" and "foods to be consumed in moderation," which are presented in the Food Purchasing Guide on page 24. The following to-be-avoided list may seem overwhelming, so concentrate on the allowed foods and the many appetizing recipes in this book that will delight your tastebuds.

Foods to be Avoided by Most

Cheese (because of tyramine, bacteria, and fermentation) You should limit all cheeses, including imitations that contain some natural cheese, except fresh cottage cheese, farmer's cheese, ricotta, and cream cheese. Avoid especially American, blue, Boursault, brick, Brie, Camembert, Cheddar, Emmentaler, Gouda, Gruyère, mozzarella, Parmesan, provolone, Roquefort, and Swiss.

Certain Beverages (because of aging, fermentation, tyramine, phenylethylamine, and caffeine) Beware of red wine, particularly Chianti, some beers and ales, liquors, cocoa, chocolate milk, excessive coffee and tea (more than two cups daily), and perhaps acidophilus milk and buttermilk.

The fermentation process in alcoholic beverages does not usually produce pressor agents, but any contamination can and often does. The protein particle, tyramine, has occurred in Chianti and byproducts of the fermentation process, called cogeners, which have been found in large amounts in Cognac and Scotch whiskeys. One sufferer rates brandy and liqueurs as the top two troublemakers, then wine, next bourbon or Scotch, and then gin. Vodka presents the least risk of all alcoholic beverages because it is pure alcohol and water.

Red wine, though, is a particularly potent migraine headache producer because it also contains histamine, which causes blood vessel reactions. Red wine is usually made with grape pulp and seeds (phenolics), which are a source of protein and can serve as a contaminant to generate blood pressor messengers. White wine and white vinegar are usually made without grape pulp or seeds and therefore may be tolerated.

Caffeine is a weak pressor agent, but in excessive amounts (more than two cups of coffee or four, 12-ounce colas daily) it may trigger a headache. Ironically, a headache may occur when excessive amounts of caffeine are suddenly stopped, as on a weekend. Theine, the stimulant in tea, affects a few people. (The caffeine content of selected foods and beverages is summarized on page 13.)

Chocolate is double trouble because in addition to caffeine it contains the naturally occurring chemical agent phenylethylamine. However, all individuals have different metabolic systems and many can tolerate cocoa, but not concentrated chocolate, as in sweets.

Some people also report headaches resulting from **rennet/milk powder pudding, yogurt, and sour cream,** so consume with caution.

Meats (because of tyramine, bacteria, and fermentation) You should avoid all aged meats and fish that are smoked, salted, pickled, or dried (such as herring and caviar) and non-fresh meats (dry and semi-dry sausages, pepperoni, salami, aged corned beef, frankfurters, ham, bologna, and cold cuts). Add to this list liver of all animals, especially chicken, liver paté, liverwurst, and goose liver.

This must-be-avoided list also includes meats that are marinated, tenderized, or aged more than 24 hours; even some cooked meats or fish that have been refrigerated more than 24 hours, such as canned tuna, sardines, or salmon, should be avoided.

Meat extracts should also be avoided because they are often concentrated from aged meats. Extracts add flavor but also contain the offending chemicals. Check food labels on gravy mixes, commercial dinners, casseroles, soups, bouillon, canned stews, etc., for meat extracts. And when eating out, choose plainer dishes rather than casseroles or dishes with sauces.

Fresh beef, lamb, poultry, and fish are non-offenders although some find pork troublesome. Snails and artificial crab have been dangerous to some.

Certain Vegetables (because of dopamine) Most vegetables are safe, but a few are definitely on the to-be-avoided lists. Fortunately, these offending triggers are not too common favorites: soy beans, Italian green beans, and broad bean pods, such as fava.

Some people also cannot freely eat legumes, such as peas, any beans, lentils, or Chinese pea pods. Definitely eliminate sauerkraut and other aged foods from your diet.

Other vegetables to be consumed with caution (1/2 cup or 4 ounces or less) are raw onions, beets (roots), and mushrooms.

Certain Fruits (because of dopamine) Most fruits are safe; however, the following may be a problem for some: avocado, ripe banana, citrus (l'octopamine), red plums, rhubarb, papaya, raisins, dried fruit, and dates. If you regularly eat more than 1/2 cup (4 ounces) of any of these, it might be advantageous to test their headache connection by avoiding them for a period of time.

Certain Additives (because of glutamine and nitrates) Monosodium glutamate (MSG), is a common additive in more than 2,000 foods and makes the to-be-avoided list because it contains glutamine, which is another chemical blood vessel messenger. Other additives that can cause headaches in some people (approximately one out of four or six, depending upon the authority) are nitrate and sodium (as in salt).

Herbert Schaumberg, M.D., isolated monosodium glutamate as a cause of headache in his report, "The Chinese Restaurant Syndrome." So many commercial products contain MSG that home prepared foods may be preferable to commercially prepared mixes and eating out. When dining in a restaurant, be sure to ask if it is possible to have your meal without MSG added.

To many people, salt-loaded foods can be a trigger. The most common offenders are not cooked foods where salt is mixed and diluted, but in highly salted items such as potato chips, nuts, crackers, pretzels, pickles, olives, anchovies, etc. Often these "appetizers" are eaten on an empty stomach; add an alcoholic drink and a previous week of stress, and you may lose a weekend to a headache.

If heavily salted foods are a headache trigger, then soy sauce, some salad dressings, Worcestershire sauce, and other such seasonings are probably headache triggers. Flavorings such as curry powder and licorice are possibilities, too, for some.

The effects of aspartame (phenylalanine), known commonly by its brand name, NutraSweet, were shown in one study to cause a significant increase in headaches for sensitive individuals. This sugar substitute is being used more and more commercially and could add up to significant amounts in the diet.

Nuts (Because of tyramine, phenylalanine, and histidine) Nuts of all varieties may be possible culprits to consider. Coconut seems to be one of the least. Peanuts and peanut butter are the most likely to trigger a headache.

Yeast (because of fermentation) The last offending agent on the to-be-avoided list is yeast. Therefore, avoid yeast extracts, yeast pills, and brewer's yeast. For some individuals, freshly baked yeast breads that are still hot, including yeast-raised doughnuts, are dangerous.

Caffeine Content of Selected Foods and Beverages

	Caffeine (mg/fl. oz.)
Coffee—roasted, ground, instant	
Percolated	8-34
Drip	11-35
Decaffeinated	0.2-0.4
Instant, decaffeinated	0.4-1.6
Instant, percolated & drip	6-35
Tea	
Bagged	6-9
Leaf	6-10
Instant	5-6
Cocoa	2-7
Soft Drinks—Regular	
Cola or Dr. Pepper	2.5-3.8
Decaffeinated cola	trace
Lemon-lime (clear)	0
Orange	0
Other citrus	0-4.5
Root beer	0
Ginger ale	0
Soft Drinks—Diet	
Cola or Dr. Pepper	0.1-4.9
Decaffeinated diet cola	trace-0.015
Diet lemon-lime	0
Diet root beer	0
Club soda, seltzer, sparkling water, tonic	0
Chocolate	
Chocolate bar, 30 g	4
Milk chocolate, 1 oz	1-15
Sweet chocolate	5-35
Chocolate milk, 8 oz	2-5
Baking chocolate, 1 oz	8-118

Caffeine, the active ingredient in coffee beans, can, in some individuals, act as a diuretic, increase blood pressure, stimulate the central nervous system, or cause other reactions. Similar, milder active ingredients are found in tea (theophylline) and in cocoa beans (theobromine).

CHAPTER THREE

Are Your Medications Causing Headaches?

IT MAY SURPRISE you that many medications, both prescription and over-the-counter, can trigger migraines either by the ingredients they contain or the medication's overall effect on the body. A reaction may also occur if medication is combined with a certain food or another medication.

Unfortunately, these medication-induced headaches are often individualized, so one drug may be helpful to some but precipitates headaches in another. These agents are many and varied, but in general may cause dilation of the blood vessels in the head.[7]

It is important that your physician knows you and your case, as well as all your medications. Together, you can identify the medications you are sensitive to, as well as the foods, so that the headache (triggering) agents are blocked.

There are many potent headache-triggers in medications, so keeping a diary of your intake of all kinds of medications, including whatever you eat or drink, may offer clues to the causes of your headaches. You may find that a headache occurs within minutes of taking an offending medication. Significant amounts of a medication may enter the bloodstream as early as five minutes after ingestion, according to John B. Brainard, M.D. As he says, "This rapid absorption into the body is logical, when one considers that nitroglycerine, an angina medication, is routinely given to patients as a tablet to be held under the tongue, where it is absorbed in a few minutes. This quick reaction accounts for the sudden onset of a headache (from certain medications), before the digestion of food which may take one-half to five hours."

Betty Brackenridge, R.D., encourages the creation of a "super" supermarket shopping plan: consider not only the offending foods, but also the offending medication purchases. Before buying or taking a medication, ask your physician or pharmacist about the ingredients and check drug labels, both those at home as well as new ones.

Although drugs will cause different reactions in different people, there are some general medications that should be checked for headache triggers:

- ❏ Sleep Aids
- ❏ Cold Medications
- ❏ Nasal Decongestants
- ❏ Cough Suppressants
- ❏ Pain Pills
- ❏ Oral Contraceptives

Specific reactive agents to look for on drug labels include caffeine, salt (sodium), propranolol, nitroglycerine, codeine, amphetamines, serotonin, MAOI inhibitors (monoamine oxidase), and licorice.

If caffeine is a headache trigger for you, then many stimulants and pain killers may cause a headache because they contain caffeine. Interestingly, some of these caffeine-containing medications effectively prevent headaches in some individuals if taken daily.

If salt (sodium) is a substance you're sensitive to, be aware that there are a host of prescription and over-the-counter medications that contain salt or sodium, such as analgesics, antacid-analgesics, antacid laxatives, and antacids. Vitamin and mineral supplements may be additional sources of sodium, so check the label! As yet, the evidence on fish oil medications is inconclusive as to their effect on headaches.

Licorice in quantity can cause sodium retention, potassium loss, diarrhea, and elevated blood pressure.

Three plants, mistletoe, viscum, and American mistletoe, should not be used in drugs (or beverages or foods) since they contain the toxic pressor B-phenylethylamine and tyramine.

Oral contraceptives may contain chemicals that decrease the brain messenger, serotonin (and its metabolites), as well as vitamin B_6. A decrease in B_6 could cause depression. Depression is relieved with a supplement of 20 to 40 milligrams of B_6 daily on a physician's advice.

Depression medications, if specifically prescribed as monoamine oxidase inhibitors, increase serotonin (tyramine) effects. So food containing tyramines should not be added to the intake.

Alcohol-sensitive individuals should beware of flavorings with high percents of alcohol; some medications, such as cough syrups, may be potent.

Finally, be wary of prescriptions containing propranolol and nitroglycerine (high blood pressure and angina medications), which affect blood vessels and blood pressure. You should also check the ingredient lists of cold prescriptions, nasal decongestants, sinus aids, asthma inhalants, cough syrups (codeine) and all types of weight reduction products.

CHAPTER FOUR

Managing Your Migraines Through Diet

THE REWARDS OF using this cookbook are many. Most importantly, the recipes and information in this book offer more freedom from headaches. It's wonderful to be in control of triggering a headache rather than having a headache control you.

More than half of these recipes are quick or easy to prepare. They have been tested and prepared by students in class laboratories, dietitians, or home economists. Each recipe has its calorie, cholesterol, fat, and sodium content listed. (In recipes with egg substitutes or eggs, the nutritional analysis is based on the egg substitute. If you use whole eggs, see page 27 for conversion values). For those migraine sufferers who become too incapacitated to cook, consider having a stockpile of selected baby foods on hand. They are nutritious, convenient, portable, easy to eat, and free from salt and additives.

Although you'll find that the 200-plus recipes in this book are perfect for the entire family, their primary benefit is that they do not include the 12 foods that should be avoided by migraine sufferers:

Foods to Avoid

1. All cheeses including "imitation," except cottage cheese, farmer's cheese, ricotta, and cream cheese.
2. All aged meats and fish that are smoked, salted, pickled, or dried (such as herring and caviar); non-fresh meats (dry or semi-dry) sausages, pepperoni, jerky, salami, hot dogs, and aged corned beef.
3. Meats chemically tenderized or marinated more than 24 hours—and even some refrigerated fresh or cooked meats within 24 hours.
4. Liver of all animals, liverwurst, liver patés.
5. Meat and hydrolyzed protein extracts such as gravy mixes and soups.
6. Fava (Italian green beans), snow peas or broad bean pods, soya beans, and soya bean paste.
7. Yeast extracts, brewer's yeast, and freshly baked hot yeast products, such as bread, rolls, doughnuts, etc.
8. Oriental soup stocks, bean paste (miso), and pickled foods (kim chee).
9. Chocolate, cocoa, and cocoa butter.
10. Sauerkraut and other aged foods.
11. Red wines such as Chianti and burgundy; sherry, vermouth, malt beverages, alcohol-free beer, and home-brews.
12. Monosodium glutamate (MSG).

As you've learned, headaches and their triggers are often individualized; a food that causes a reaction in one person may not in another. The following foods, while not automatic headache triggers, may be dangerous to some individuals. Because the effects of these foods are not clear-cut, we have included them in some recipes. However, as you will see, they are clearly marked in each recipe so you can omit them or skip the recipe altogether. Cooking does not usually eliminate triggering agents!

Foods Dangerous to Some Individuals

(Marked with an asterisk in the recipes.)

Coffee, tea, and other caffeine-containing beverages

Salad dressing (check label for triggers)

Rennet tablets

Raisins, dried fruits, and dates

Imitation crab

Coconut

Ham, bacon, pork

Licorice

Mushrooms

Snails

Salty foods

Rhubarb

Hydrolyzed vegetable protein (check labels)

Some hard liquors and liqueurs

Vanilla and other flavorings, especially if they contain a high
   percentage of alcohol

Dried fruits, such as raisins, apricots, dates, etc., are not usually troublesome if fresh. Therefore, avoid the aged, hard, and perhaps fermented fruit products. Some individuals also report sensitivity to aspartame, milk, and vitamin-C preparations including multi-vitamin pills (if sensitive to citrus fruits).

Foods to Be Consumed with Caution

(Marked with two asterisks in the recipes.)

A third category of headache-triggering foods is those that simply should be consumed with caution. You may or may not have a reaction to the following foods. The most common are onions and lemons, which are used the world over to enhance flavor. However, if used in amounts less than 1/2 cup, they usually can be successfully tolerated by the headache-prone.

Soups made with instant soup powders

Citrus fruit, particularly orange juice, perhaps lemon

Soy sauce

Ripe avocado

Banana, particularly overripe

Yogurt, sour cream, acidophilus milk, and buttermilk
Fresh raspberries
Peanuts and some other nuts, except macadamia
Distilled spirits, including white wine
Red plums
Onions, raw, cooked, dried
Worcestershire sauce

The most definitive way of dealing with your diet is to first eat nothing that should be avoided. Then, try avoiding all foods on the second and third lists for a period of time in which you would expect to have three or more headaches. If your strategy appears to be successful, you may want to re-introduce certain favorite items such as bananas or white wine, one or two things at a time, in an attempt to broaden your diet. Return of headache or the warning signs should be fair notice to discontinue suspect items immediately.

In general, allow three days between headaches before introducing a new ingredient (agent) for testing. And read labels no matter how many times you buy a food product. Manufacturers sometimes change ingredients without warning.

As you become more familiar with your recipes and the foods to avoid, you'll find yourself able to organize and prepare many meals of excellent variety and delectable taste for yourself and others. You'll also be able to shop faster and plan and prepare meals faster.

Now, here's how to begin: Read the Food Purchasing Guide on page 24. This is an excellent guide in helping you make your food purchases. Make a copy of it and take it with you when shopping. Avoid the offending foods listed, and buy foods that are in the "foods allowed" column.

To help you keep your headache control planning simple, meal plans are provided starting on page 25. Recipes for many of the foods in the meal plans are included in this book. You can mix or match as you desire, depending on which foods you especially enjoy. The main thing to remember is to record what you've eaten, so you can quickly identify a food that triggered a headache. (That's always easier if you follow a meal plan.)

Photocopy the chart appears on the next page and use it to record your weekly intake.

Food Intake Plan and Record

WEEK OF: _____

Monday	Tuesday	Wednesday	Thursday	Friday	Saturday	Sunday
Headache(s)	Headache(s)	Headache(s)	Headache(s)	Headache(s)	Headache(s)	Headache(s)
Time(s)	Time(s)	Time(s)	Time(s)	Time(s)	Time(s)	Time(s)

Reproduction of this chart is permitted.

Food Purchasing Guide

	Foods Allowed	Foods Dangerous to Some/Consume with Caution	Foods to Avoid
Breads, Cereals, and Grain Products	Most breads; cooked and cold cereals; muffins; pancakes; waffles; cookies and cakes made without chocolate	Ready-to-eat cereals or crackers with nuts, coconut, or dried fruits; high-salt or -sodium products; some commercial mixes	Bakery and cereal products with chocolate; questionable foods if sensitive; crackers with cheese; MSG; freshly baked hot yeast products
Fruits	Any others not listed	Dried fruits, ripe banana, avocado, red plums, fresh raspberries, rhubarb, oranges, lemons, or more than one citrus daily	Any of the fruits in question in the canned state if the fresh fruit triggers a migraine
Vegetables, Legumes and Nuts	Any others not listed	Raw and cooked onions, beets, eggplant, pickled vegetables, most nuts	Broad bean pods, Italian bean pods, soya bean paste, kim chee Chinese pea pods, sauerkraut, some beans and lentils
Meat, Poultry, and Fish	Canned tuna in water; fresh beef, lamb, veal, poultry, or fish	Heavily salted canned fish, pork, ham, bacon, snails, imitation crab	All aged meats including salted, smoked, dried, pickled, marinated, or tenderized meats; sausage; pepperoni; hot togs corned beef; liver and meat extracts; patés
Milk and Dairy Products	Whole, lowfat, and skim milk, cottage cheese, ricotta cheese, cream cheese	Yogurt, sour cream, acidophilus milk, buttermilk, (1/4 to 1/2 cup depending on age and manufacturing process)	Chocolate milk; aged cheese of all kinds, natural or imitation
Fats and Oils	Any others not listed	Salad dressings and mayonnaise with wine vinegar, salt, or additives	
Alcoholic Beverages	White wine, vodka (if tolerated or desired)		Beer, ale, red wines, Chianti, sherry, vermouth, distilled liquor, liqueurs
Other	White vinegar, eggs, hard candy, vanilla ice cream, non-cola soft drinks, tapioca	Soy sauce; extracts; Worcestershire sauce; licorice; all beverages that contain caffeine; hydrolized vegetable protein; nitrites; nitrates; bouillon cubes; aspertame	Chocolate and products containing chocolate; marinades and tenderizers; yeast extracts and brewer's yeast; all aged foods; pickled foods

Meal Plan Guide

Breakfast	Lunch	Dinner	Snack
Breakfast Burrito Kiwi	**Egg Salad Sandwich** Peas with Jicama	**Stir-Fry Chicken & Broccoli** (no MSG or soy sauce) Rice, Salad	**Caramel Custard**
Jam Toast Triangles	**Chicken Pot Pie**	**Pasta Primavera with Salmon**	**Fudge Brownies**
Oatmeal and Milk Sliced Peaches	**Savory Beef Burger** Creamed Corn Relishes	**Texas Meat Loaf** Baked Potato, Salad Steamed Carrots	Pear
French Toast Strawberries	**Taco Salad** Vegetable	**Turkey "Sausage" Patties** Mixed Salad Greens **Italian Dressing**	**Poppy Seed Loaf**
Cottage Cheese on an English Muffin	**Chicken Vegetable Salad** Asparagus	**Shrimp Sauté with Dijon Mustard** **Fruit Blintz**	**Health Nog**
Omelet Primavera Half a grapefruit	Tuna Salad in a Tomato **Crunchy Bread Sticks**	**Favorite "Ham" Loaf** **Harlequin Slaw** **Pumpkin Bread**	**Lemon Love Notes**
Rice puffs and milk Melon	**Turkey Chili,** Salad **Whole Grain Muffins**	Beef Steak, Vegetable **Wild Rice Casserole**	**Sweet Potato Chips**

Items listed in **bold** are recipes in this book.

Tyramine-Restricted Diet (MAO)

Suggested Meal Plan	Sample Menu	Southwestern Menu
Breakfast		
Fruit Juice	Kiwi Fruit	Cranberry Apple Juice
Cereal	Cream of Wheat	Oatmeal
Meat/Meat Substitute	Soft Cooked Egg	Soft Cooked Egg with Salsa
Bread with margarine	Toast with butter or margarine	Tortilla with butter or margarine
Milk	Milk	Milk
Beverage	Coffee or Tea	Coffee or Tea
Lunch		
Meat/Meat Substitute	Broiled Beef Patty	Boiled Pinto Beans with Salsa
Potato/Potato Substitute	Mashed Potatoes	Rice
Vegetable and/or Salad	Steamed Spinach	Steamed Spinach
Dessert	Gelatin Cubes	Flan (caramel custard)
Bread with margarine	Whole Wheat Bread with margarine	Flour Tortilla
Beverage	Coffee or Tea	Coffee or Tea
Dinner		
Soup or Juice	Consommé	Broth
Meat/Meat Substitute	Roast Chicken	Roast Chicken
Vegetable and/or Salad	Peas	Peas
Bread with margarine	Creamy Coleslaw	Creamy Coleslaw
Dessert	Biscuit with margarine	Flour Tortilla
Milk	Baked Apple	Fresh Apple
Beverage	Milk	Milk
	Coffee or Tea	Coffee or Tea

Nutrient Analysis of Tyramine-Restricted Sample Menu

Calories	1700
Vitamin A	1371 RE
Calcium	952 mg
Iron	13 mg
Dietary Fiber	16 gm
Folate	337 mg
Protein	102 gm
Vitamin C	99 mg
Phosphorus	1493 mg
Sodium	2373 mg
Cholesterol	443 mg
Thiamin	1.3 mg
Carbohydrate	176 gm
Niacin	25 mg
Zinc	12 mg
Potassium	3040 mg
Fat	68 gm
Riboflavin	1.9 mg

Adapted from *Arizona Diet Manual* by Ann Moore Allan

Nutritional Content
of Four Recipe Ingredients

FAT	Calories	Salt	Cholesterol	Fat
Butter (1 Tbsp.)	102	95 mg	33 mg	11.5 g
Margarine (1 Tbsp.)	102	95 mg	—	11.5 g
Soft Stick (1 Tbsp.)	80	79 mg	—	8 g
Vegetable Oil (1 Tbsp.)	120	70 mg	—	13.6 g
Cooking Spray (1 1/2 sec.)	7	0	0	1 g
EGGS				
Egg Substitute (1/4 c.)	25	80 mg	0 mg	0 g
Egg (1 whole)	70	60 mg	240 mg	5 g
MILK				
Whole (1 cup - 4%)	157	119 mg	35 mg	8.9 g
2% (1 cup)	121	122 mg	18 mg	4.7 g
1% (1 cup)	102	123 mg	10 mg	2.6 g
Skim (1 cup)	86	126 mg	4 mg	.4 g
Buttermilk (1 cup)	99	257 mg	9 mg	2.2 g

SALT	Sodium	Potassium
Salt (1 tsp.)	2300 mg	0
Garlic Salt (1 tsp.)	2050 mg	Trace
Butter-Flavored (1 tsp.)	1125 mg	0
Season All (1 tsp.)	980 mg	17 mg
Lite Salt (1 tsp.	1100 mg	1500 mg
No Salt (1 tsp.)	1500 mg	385 mg

PART TWO

Recipes

(Migraine-Proofed)

Appetizers
& Beverages

Chicken Paté

Here's a paté minus the liver, that you can indulge in to your heart's content.

Specialty

Onion**

1-1/2 pounds boneless uncooked CHICKEN BREASTS, ground
1 cup finely chopped, peeled APPLE
1 cup dry BREAD CRUMBS
1/2 cup finely chopped ONION**
1/2 cup EGG SUBSTITUTE or 2 EGGS
3 Tbsp. MARGARINE
3 Tbsp. WHITE VINEGAR
1/2 tsp. THYME LEAVES
1/2 tsp. BASIL LEAVES
1/4 tsp. crushed fresh GARLIC
1/8 tsp. PEPPER

Preheat oven to 350 degrees. Thoroughly combine ground chicken, apple, bread crumbs, onion, eggs or egg substitute, 2 tablespoons margarine, vinegar, thyme, basil, garlic, and pepper. Grease a loaf pan (8 1/2 x 4 1/2 x 2 1/2) with 2 teaspoons margarine. Press chicken mixture into pan. Dot with remaining margarine. Set loaf pan in shallow pan of water and bake for one hour or until firm and pulling away from sides of pan. Drain excess liquid from pan. Cover and weight down paté while it is very hot. Cool slightly and then refrigerate, weighted, until well chilled.

MICROWAVE: Prepare chicken mixture as above, using a 5-cup microwave-safe ring mold. Cover. Microwave on high (100% power) for 6 to 8 minutes, rotating 1/2 turn after 3 minutes. Weight and chill as above.

MAKES ONE LOAF (32 SERVINGS)
SERVING SIZE: 1/8" SLICE
CALORIES: 50 • CHOL.: 12 MG. • FAT: 1 G. • SODIUM: 42 MG.

---

*=Dangerous to some • **=Consume with caution • See pages 19-22 for more information

Cucumber Canapés

A bright and colorful, crunchy canapé that is also cholesterol-lowering.

Specialty

Onion**

> 1/4 cup MARGARINE, softened
> 1 tsp. grated ONION**
> 24 (2 inch) BREAD ROUNDS
> 24 slices CUCUMBER
> 2 Tbsp. CREAMY MAYONNAISE (see Salads)
> 3 Tbsp. chopped PARSLEY
> 6 CHERRY TOMATOES, thinly sliced

In small bowl, blend together margarine and onion. Spread rounds of bread with mixture. Top each with a cucumber slice and 1/4 teaspoon Creamy Mayonnaise. Garnish with parsley and a tomato slice.

MAKES 2 DOZEN
SERVING SIZE: 1 CANAPÉ
CALORIES: 41 • CHOL.: 0 • FAT: 2 G. • SODIUM: 53 MG.

Sweet Potato Chips

These are delicious and flavorful and an excellent source of the vegetable form of vitamin "A," beta carotene.

Specialty

> 2 cups very thinly sliced SWEET POTATOES
> 2 tsp. BUTTER
> 1 Tbsp. BROWN SUGAR

Spread potato slices in microwave-safe dish. Sprinkle with water. Microwave on high 5 minutes. Mix butter and brown sugar and spread on slices. Microwave another 2 to 5 minutes. Let stand until cool.

MAKES 4 SERVINGS
SERVING SIZE: 1/2 CUP
CALORIES: 59 • CHOL.: 5 MG. • FAT: 2 G. • SODIUM: 21 MG.

*=Dangerous to some • **=Consume with caution • See pages 19-22 for more information

Individual Salmon Soufflés

Here's a healthy version for entertaining that's really different.
This dish takes a bit of time, but it's well worth the effort.

Specialty

Scallions, Lemon juice****

SINGLE CRUST FLAKY PASTRY, doubled (see Desserts)
1-1/4 cups SKIM MILK
1/4 cup quick-cooking TAPIOCA
1/4 cup EGG SUBSTITUTE or 1 EGG
1 Tbsp. MARGARINE
1/2 pound RED SALMON, poached in water
2 Tbsp. finely chopped SCALLIONS**
2 Tbsp. minced PARSLEY
1 Tbsp. LEMON JUICE**
1/2 tsp. DRY MUSTARD
1/8 tsp. PEPPER
4 EGG WHITES, stiffly beaten

Preheat oven to 400 degrees. Roll pastry into 16 (4-inch) circles. Mold on bottom and sides of muffin cups to make shells. Prick pastry with a fork and bake for 10 minutes or until golden brown. Remove to wire racks to cool.

Combine skim milk, tapioca, and egg substitute; let stand for 5 minutes. Bring to a boil; cook and stir until very thick, about 10 minutes. Remove from heat; stir in margarine.

Skin and bone poached salmon; flake meat. Combine salmon, scallions, parsley, lemon juice, mustard, and pepper thoroughly; blend in cooked tapioca mixture. Stir 1/3 beaten egg whites into salmon mixture. Fold in remaining beaten egg whites. Spoon into pastry shells, mounding tops. Place on baking sheet; bake at 350 degrees for 30 to 35 minutes or until puffed and golden brown. Serve immediately.

MAKES 16 APPETIZERS
SERVING SIZE: 1 APPETIZER
CALORIES: 190 • CHOL.: 9 MG. • FAT: 9 G. • SODIUM: 105 MG

*=Dangerous to some • **=Consume with caution • See pages 19-22 for more information

Spinach Balls

This unusual recipe can be served as a terrifically tasty appetizer or as a great evening snack!

Quick and Easy • Prepare Ahead

Onion**

1 pkg. (10 oz.) frozen CHOPPED SPINACH, thawed and squeezed dry
1 cup HERBED SEASONED STUFFING MIX
1 small ONION**, chopped
3/4 cup EGG SUBSTITUTE, or 3 eggs
1 Tbsp. MARGARINE, melted

Preheat oven to 350 degrees. In medium bowl, combine spinach, stuffing mix, and onion. Blend in egg substitute and melted margarine. Shape into 1-inch balls. Place on lightly greased baking sheet. Bake for 10 to 15 minutes. Serve hot.

MICROWAVE: Prepare as above. Arrange 12 balls in 9-inch microwave-safe pie plate. Microwave on high (100% power) for 2-1/2 to 3 minutes. Rotate dish 1/2 turn after 1-1/2 minutes. Repeat with remaining spinach balls.

TIP: Prepare ahead. May be wrapped and frozen, then reheated and served later.

MAKES 36 SPINACH BALLS
SERVING SIZE: 1 SPINACH BALL
CALORIES: 12 • CHOL.: 0 • FAT: 1 G. • SODIUM: 33 MG.

Tortilla "Chips" & Low-Fat "Guacamole" Dip

Enjoy this low-fat dip without guilt!

Quick and Easy

Lime juice**

NONSTICK COOKING SPRAY
10 CORN TORTILLAS, cut into wedges
SALT or SALT SUBSTITUTE, if tolerated
2 cups condensed GREEN SPLIT PEA SOUP, chilled
1 tsp. LIME JUICE**
1 small TOMATO, seeds removed
1/8 tsp. GARLIC POWDER or 1 fine minced GARLIC clove
1 can (4 oz.) chopped GREEN CHILES
1 Tbsp. chunky SALSA (mild, medium, or hot)
TABASCO® to taste
GREEN FOOD COLORING

Preheat oven to 350 degrees. Cut corn tortillas into wedges, spray with cooking spray and bake for 8 to 10 minutes or until crisp. Sprinkle chips with light salt or salt substitute, if tolerated.

Combine the rest of the ingredients except Tabasco and food coloring in food processor or blender. Blend well until smooth and creamy. Add a drop of coloring, one at a time, until nice and green. Add Tabasco to taste.

PREPARE AHEAD TIP: Flavors enhance and dip holds well if prepared 2 to 6 hours ahead and refrigerated.

MAKES 2-1/2 CUPS (40 TBSP.)
SERVING SIZE: 1 TBSP.
CALORIES: 15 • CHOL: 0 • FAT: .05 G. • SODIUM: 62 MG.

Stuffed Mushrooms

You might want to consider this appetizer as part of an hors d'oeuvre platter when company calls. The walnuts are not usually a trigger agent nor is the small amount of onion.

Specialty

Mushrooms*, Onion**, Walnuts**

18 medium MUSHROOMS*, fresh
2 Tbsp. MARGARINE
1/4 cup chopped ONIONS**, minced
1 clove GARLIC, minced
1/2 cup WALNUTS**, chopped
1/4 cup fresh BREAD CRUMBS
1 Tbsp. PARSLEY, chopped
1/4 tsp. BLACK PEPPER
dash RED PEPPER

Preheat oven to 350 degrees. Remove stems from mushrooms. Chop stems and set aside. Melt margarine in skillet. Mix in chopped mushroom stems, onion, and garlic; sauté until tender. Mix in walnuts, bread crumbs, parsley, black pepper, and red pepper. Place mushroom caps on broiler rack. Stuff each cap with prepared filling. Bake for 15 to 20 minutes or until done.

MICROWAVE: Remove stems from mushrooms; chop stems and set aside. In 1-1/2 quart microwave-proof casserole, microwave chopped stems, margarine, onion, garlic, and walnuts on high (100% power) for 2 to 2-1/2 minutes, stirring once. Stir in bread crumbs, parsley, black pepper, and red pepper; stuff mushroom caps. Arrange stuffed mushrooms, 9 at a time, on a paper plate. Microwave on high for 2 to 3 minutes, rotating 1/2 turn after 1-1/2 minutes. Repeat with remaining mushrooms.

MAKES 1-1/2 DOZEN APPETIZERS
SERVING SIZE: 1 STUFFED MUSHROOM
CALORIES: 43 • CHOL.: 0 • FAT: 3 G. • SODIUM: 15 MG.

Nippy Dip

High in calcium and can also be used as a sandwich spread!

Prepare Ahead • Quick and Easy

Green onion**,Lemon juice**,Yogurt**

1 cup LOW-FAT COTTAGE CHEESE
3 Tbsp. finely chopped fresh PARSLEY
1/4 tsp. dried whole DILLWEED
3 Tbsp. reduced-calorie MAYONNAISE (check label)
SALT or SALT SUBSTITUTE to taste
3 Tbsp. minced GREEN ONIONS**
1/2 tsp. LEMON JUICE**
1/2 cup PLAIN NONFAT YOGURT**

Combine cottage cheese and remaining ingredients in a bowl or blender; mix well. Cover and chill 3 hours. Serve with carrot and celery sticks or plain crackers.

PREPARE AHEAD TIP: Flavors enhance and dip holds well if prepared 3 to 6 hours ahead and refrigerated.

MAKES 1-3/4 CUPS
SERVING SIZE: 1 TBSP.
CALORIES: 13 • CHOL.: 1 MG. • FAT: 0.5 G. • SODIUM: 48 MG.

Red, White & Green Dip

Perfect for Christmas or any holiday.

Quick and Easy • Prepare Ahead

Onion**, Chives**

12 oz. LOW-FAT COTTAGE CHEESE
1 Tbsp. chopped RED PEPPER or PIMENTO
1/4 cup chopped ONION**
pinch of SALT and PEPPER
1 Tbsp. chopped CHIVES**
1 Tbsp. chopped GREEN PEPPER
1/2 cup SKIM MILK
PAPRIKA

Mix all ingredients except skim milk and paprika. Thin with the milk to desired consistency. Sprinkle with paprika.

PREPARE AHEAD TIP: Flavors are enhanced if prepared 2 to 6 hours ahead and refrigerated.

MAKES 2 CUPS
SERVING SIZE: 1-1/2 TBSP.
CALORIES: 14 • CHOL.: 1 MG. • FAT: 0 • SODIUM: 4 MG.

Salsa Dip

A southwestern dip to scoop up with tortilla or corn chips.

Quick and Easy

Onion**, Lime juice**

1 CUCUMBER, diced
3 TOMATILLOS (broil and remove skins)
1 Tbsp. WHITE VINEGAR
JUICE of 1 LIME**
1 tsp. chopped JALAPEÑO PEPPER
1 TOMATO, chopped
1 Tbsp. chopped RED ONION**
pinch of SALT SUBSTITUTE, if tolerated

Combine all ingredients in blender or food processor. Pulse until chunky.

MAKES 1-1/2 CUPS
SERVING SIZE: 1 TBSP.
CALORIES: 6 • CHOL.: 0 • FAT: 1 G. • SODIUM: 2 MG.

Coffee Variations

If coffee is not a trigger for you, or decaf is safe, try these variations for a delicious drink.

Quick and Easy

Coffee*, Orange rind**

Hot Spiced Coffee

2/3 cup 2% low-fat MILK
1 Tbsp. BROWN SUGAR
1/4 tsp. GROUND ALLSPICE
1 (4-inch) strip ORANGE RIND**
1 (3-inch) STICK CINNAMON, crushed
3-1/2 cups hot brewed COFFEE*

Combine milk, brown sugar, allspice, orange rind, and cinnamon in a saucepan; bring to a boil. Remove from heat, and let stand 5 minutes. Line a colander with 4 layers of cheesecloth, allowing cheesecloth to extend over outside edges. Place colander over a large bowl or pitcher. Pour milk mixture into colander; discard spices. Add coffee to milk mixture; stir well. Serve immediately. Makes 4 cups.

Spiced Iced Coffee

Pour 3 cups of hot, double-strength coffee over 2 cinnamon sticks, 4 cloves, and 4 allspice berries. Let stand 1 hour; strain. Pour over ice in four tall glasses.

Coffee Julep

Just add a dash of mint flavor to your iced coffee and serve in silver or aluminum tumblers, well frosted.

NOTE: Hot Spiced Coffee contains 33 calories per cup; 25 mg. sodium; and 3 mg. cholesterol.

---

*=Dangerous to some • **=Consume with caution • See pages 19-22 for more information

Cranberry Cooler

A wonderfully refreshing drink that's beneficial as well!

Quick and Easy

Lemon juice**

1/4 cup CRANAPPLE JUICE or use CRANBERRY or other CRANBERRY JUICE BLENDS
3/4 cup CLUB SODA
1 tsp. LEMON JUICE**
1/2 cup CRUSHED ICE

Combine cranapple juice, club soda, and lemon juice. Stir and pour over crushed ice.

TIP: Team cooler with up to 3 cups "light" microwave popcorn or another low-fat snack. Check the package label for brands of popcorn that contain up to 2 grams or less of fat per 1 cup serving (to reduce calories).

MAKES 1 SERVING
SERVING SIZE: 1 CUP
CALORIES: 42 • CHOL.: 0 • FAT: 1 G. • SODIUM: 1 MG.

Creamy Mint Shake

Such a refreshing summer treat!

Quick and Easy

Yogurt**

1/2 cup CRUSHED ICE
1/4 cup SPARKLING MINERAL WATER
1 (8 oz.) carton VANILLA LOW-FAT YOGURT** or ice-milk dessert
1 tsp. SUGAR
1/4 cup lightly packed fresh MINT LEAVES
fresh MINT LEAVES (optional)

Combine ice, mineral water, yogurt, sugar, and mint leaves in blender; cover and process 1 minute or until smooth. Serve immediately. Garnish with mint.

MAKES 2 SERVINGS
SERVING SIZE: 1 CUP
CALORIES: 107 • CHOL.: 6 MG. • FAT: 1.4 G. • SODIUM: 84 MG.

Health Nog

*Almost a complete meal that tastes luscious
and is luscious for your nutritional needs, too.*

Quick and Easy

Orange juice**

10 fresh or frozen STRAWBERRIES (if using frozen, let partially thaw)
3 cups SKIM MILK
1 cup EGG SUBSTITUTE
1/3 cup frozen ORANGE JUICE CONCENTRATE**
1/4 cup HONEY
1 Tbsp. WHEAT GERM (optional)

Place strawberries in bowl or blender/food processor. Mix or blend until smooth. Add skim milk, egg substitute, orange juice concentrate, honey, and wheat germ (if desired). Mix or blend until well combined. Serve immediately.

MAKES 8 SERVINGS
SERVING SIZE: 3/4 CUP
CALORIES: 106 • CHOL.: 4 • FAT: 1 G. • SODIUM: 93 MG.

L'Orange Refresher

Use only 1/3 cup of ingredients that are dangerous for you.

Quick and Easy

Orange juice**, Banana**, Yogurt**

1/2 cup ORANGE or PINEAPPLE JUICE**
1/4 cup 100% BRAN CEREAL
1/2 medium ripe BANANA**
1/2 cup PLAIN NONFAT YOGURT**
1/4 cup SKIM MILK

Place all ingredients in bowl or blender/food processor. Mix or blend until smooth. If using mixer, let bran soak in liquids for a few minutes first. Serve immediately.

NOTE: This drink does have 3 possible headache triggers for some individuals. Reducing the 1/2 cup measure to 1/3 cup may prevent a reaction, or simply delete if the item is aged.

MAKES 1 SERVING
SERVING SIZE: 1-1/4 CUPS
CALORIES: 264 • CHOL.: 9 MG. • FAT: 3 G. • SODIUM: 282 MG.

Skim Milk Hot "Cocoa"

With carob powder it almost tastes like chocolate!

Quick and Easy

Vanilla*

2 Tbsp. CAROB POWDER
3 Tbsp. SUGAR or ARTIFICIAL SWEETENER
1/4 cup HOT WATER
1-1/2 cups SKIM MILK
1/8 tsp. VANILLA EXTRACT*

In small saucepan blend carob powder and sugar; gradually add hot water. Cook over medium heat, stirring constantly, until mixture boils; boil and stir for 2 minutes. Add milk; heat thoroughly. Stir occasionally; do not boil. Remove from heat; add vanilla. Serve hot.

MAKES 2 SERVINGS
SERVING SIZE: 7 OUNCES
CALORIES: 161 • CHOL.: 3 MG. • FAT: 1 G. • SODIUM: 97 MG.

Soups, Salads, & Salad Dressings

Double Potato Soup

This different version of potato soup can be made a main course by adding diced chicken breast and serving with crusty French bread and fruit. This recipe will give you enough to freeze for another meal.

Prepare Ahead

Onion**

1 Tbsp. MARGARINE
1 medium YELLOW ONION**, chopped
2 cans (14.5 oz. each) CHICKEN BROTH
4 cups WATER
4 large WHITE BAKING POTATOES, diced
1 large SWEET POTATO, peeled and diced
1/8 tsp. PEPPER
1 Tbsp. DILL WEED

Melt margarine in a large soup pot. Add onion; cook over medium-low heat for 10 minutes. Add broth, water, potatoes, and sweet potato. Bring to boil; reduce heat to medium-low and cook for about 20 minutes, or until potatoes are tender.

Remove soup from heat. When cool, puree liquids and solids in a blender or food processor (do in 3 batches). Return puree to pot. If consistency is too thick, add water until soup reaches desired consistency. Add pepper and dill. Keep warm over low heat.

MAKES 12 SERVINGS
SERVING SIZE: 1 CUP
CALORIES: 73 • CHOL.: 5 MG. • FAT: 5 G. • SODIUM: 1,000 MG.

Egg Drop Soup

Quick and Easy

Scallions**

4 cups WATER
4 packets or cubes low-sodium CHICKEN BOUILLON
3 Tbsp. CORNSTARCH
1/4 tsp. TARRAGON LEAVES
3 Tbsp. EGG SUBSTITUTE, or 1 whole EGG, beaten
2 SCALLIONS**, finely chopped

In medium saucepan, bring 3-1/2 cups water to a boil. Stir in chicken bouillon until dissolved. Combine cornstarch and remaining 1/2 cup water; add to bouillon, stirring constantly. Mix in tarragon. Cook and stir until thickened and boiling. Cook 1 minute longer. Reduce heat to low; gradually add egg substitute or beaten egg in a thin stream, without stirring. Cook for 30 seconds. Stir once or twice. Serve in bowls garnished with scallions.

MAKES 6 SERVINGS
SERVING SIZE: 3/4 CUP
CALORIES: 28 • CHOL.: 0 • FAT: 0 • SODIUM: 17 MG.

---

*=Dangerous to some • **=Consume with caution • See pages 19-22 for more information

Cabbage Soup

Quick and Easy

Onion**

6 cups CABBAGE, chopped (or use pre-shredded cabbage)
1/4 tsp. CARAWAY SEED
1/8 tsp. PEPPER
1-1/2 tsp. SALT (optional)
1/4 tsp. DILL WEED
1 medium ONION**, peeled, sliced, and separated into rings
4 cups hot WATER

Combine all ingredients; cover, and simmer 15 to 20 minutes until cabbage and onion are tender.

MAKES 6 SERVINGS
SERVING SIZE: 1 CUP
CALORIES: 59 • CHOL: 0 • FAT: 0 • SODIUM: 142 MG

Creamy Romano Tomato Soup

Remember when your mother brought you this comforting, tasty soup? Now yours is homemade and even better!

Quick and Easy

1-3/4 cups whole peeled ROMANO TOMATOES, (14-1/2 oz. can), undrained
2/3 cup (6 oz. can) TOMATO PASTE
1 cup LOW-FAT MILK
1/2 cup low-salt canned CHICKEN BROTH or 1 BOUILLON CUBE
fresh BASIL SPRIGS

In blender or food processor, process tomatoes and juice, and tomato paste until blended. Stir in milk and chicken broth. Pour through sieve into medium saucepan to remove tomato seeds. Heat to serving temperature. Garnish with fresh basil.

MAKES 4 SERVINGS
SERVING SIZE: 1 CUP
CALORIES: 106 • CHOL.: 5 MG. • FAT: 1 G. • SODIUM: 350 G.

Lemon Soup

Quick and Easy

Lemon juice**

2 cans (14.5 oz. each) CHICKEN BROTH
2 cups cooked WHITE RICE
1-1/2 cups WATER
1 cup EGG SUBSTITUTE, or 4 EGGS, beaten
1/4 cup LEMON JUICE**
1 pkg. (10 oz.) FROZEN SPINACH, thawed and drained
1/8 tsp. PEPPER

Pour broth into pot and bring to a boil. Add rice and water. Simmer 2 minutes. Combine egg substitute and lemon juice in a small bowl and mix well. Remove soup from heat.

Mix 2 cups of hot broth into egg mixture, stirring constantly. Pour mixture back into broth; stir in spinach. Add pepper; simmer for 5 minutes.

MAKES 6 SERVINGS
SERVING SIZE: 1 CUP
CALORIES: 126 • CHOL.: 2 MG. • FAT: 1 G. • SODIUM: 364 MG.

Mac & Beef Soup

This soup is really a complete meal, yet easy to make, and even better the second time around—but not over 24 hours!

Prepare Ahead

Onion**, Lemon juice**

NONSTICK COOKING SPRAY
1/2 lb. lean GROUND BEEF
1/2 cup chopped GREEN PEPPER
1/2 cup chopped ONION**
1/2 tsp. dried OREGANO LEAVES, crushed
1/2 tsp. dried BASIL LEAVES, crushed
3 cans (10-3/4 oz. each) TOMATO SOUP
3 soup cans WATER
2 cups ELBOW MACARONI, cooked in unsalted water and drained
2 tsp. LEMON JUICE**

Spray 6-quart pan with cooking spray. Over medium heat, cook beef, green pepper, and onion with oregano and basil until beef is browned and vegetables are tender, stirring to separate meat. Spoon off fat.

Stir in soup, water, macaroni, and lemon juice. Heat to boiling. Reduce heat to low. Simmer 20 minutes, stirring occasionally.

MAKES 8 SERVINGS
SERVING SIZE: 1-1/3 CUPS
CALORIES: 180 • CHOL.: 21 MG. • FAT: 3 G. • SODIUM: 367 MG.

Gazpacho

For hot summer days this southwestern soup is a natural; the green peppers, tomatoes, and tomato juice contribute valuable vitamin C for summer stress.

Specialty

Onion**, Lemon juice**

3/4 cup TOMATO JUICE

2 Tbsp. LEMON JUICE**

3 Tbsp. SPICY TOMATO DRESSING (see Salads)

2 Tbsp. finely chopped CELERY

1/4 tsp. GARLIC POWDER

1 Tbsp. chopped PARSLEY

3 cups fat-free BEEF BROTH or BOUILLON CUBES

1/3 cup finely chopped ONIONS**

1/3 cup finely chopped GREEN PEPPERS

1 cup diced, peeled, and cored fresh TOMATOES

1 tsp. SALT or SALT SUBSTITUTE

1/4 to 1/2 cup thinly sliced or diced CUCUMBERS

Combine all ingredients except cucumbers in a large bowl. Mix gently and refrigerate at least 4 hours. Garnish with cucumbers before serving.

MAKES 5 SERVINGS

SERVING SIZE: 3/4 CUP

CALORIES: 35 • CHOL.: 0 • FAT: 1 G. • SODIUM: 944 MG.

Turkey Minestrone

An old-fashioned, satisfying soup for a meal in itself. If any is left over, fill plastic drinking glasses, cover, and freeze for individual servings with sandwiches another time.

Quick and Easy • Prepare Ahead

Onion**

NONSTICK COOKING SPRAY
1 pkg. (about 1-1/4 lb.) fresh lean GROUND TURKEY
2 cups shredded CABBAGE
1 cup sliced CARROTS
1/2 cup chopped ONION**
1-1/2 tsp. dried BASIL LEAVES
1/4 tsp. GARLIC POWDER
1/4 tsp. PEPPER
3 cans (14-1/2 oz. each) reduced-sodium or regular BEEF BROTH
1 can (16 oz.) whole TOMATOES, undrained, cut up
1 medium ZUCCHINI, diced
1 pkg. (9 oz.) frozen cut GREEN BEANS
chopped fresh PARSLEY, if desired

Spray bottom of 6-quart saucepan or Dutch oven with nonstick cooking spray until well coated. Heat saucepan over medium-high heat about 30 seconds. Crumble ground turkey into pan. Cook and stir 3 to 5 minutes or until lightly browned. Add cabbage, carrots, onion, basil, garlic powder, pepper, beef broth, and tomatoes; bring to a boil. Reduce heat to medium; cook 10 minutes, stirring occasionally. Add zucchini and green beans; cook an additional 8 to 12 minutes or until vegetables are tender, stirring occasionally. Sprinkle with chopped fresh parsley, if desired.

MAKES 8 SERVINGS
SERVING SIZE: 1-1/2 CUPS
CALORIES: 160 • CHOL.: 48 MG. • FAT: 6 G. • SODIUM: 145 MG.

*=Dangerous to some • **=Consume with caution • See pages 19-22 for more information

Simple Hot & Sour Soup

You may have seen this favorite on Chinese menus.
Try it in your own kitchen for a change.

Quick and Easy

Mushrooms*, Onions**, Lemon juice**

1 tsp. SESAME OIL
1/2 medium ONION**, finely chopped
2-1/2 cans (14.5 oz. each) CHICKEN BROTH
1 Tbsp. LEMON JUICE**
1 Tbsp. TABASCO SAUCE
1 Tbsp. WHITE VINEGAR
1 can (6 oz.) WATER CHESTNUTS
1/2 cup LOW-FAT COTTAGE CHEESE
3 dried MUSHROOMS*, soaked in cold water for 10 minutes and chopped
2 Tbsp. CORNSTARCH
2 Tbsp. cold WATER
1/4 cup EGG SUBSTITUTE, or 1 EGG, beaten
1 GREEN ONION**, finely chopped

Heat oil in a saucepan. Add onions and cook until soft. Gradually add broth. Stir in lemon juice, Tabasco sauce, vinegar, chestnuts, cottage cheese, and mushrooms. Simmer for 15 minutes. Bring to boil. Mix cornstarch and water, and add to boiling soup; stir until thickened. Add egg substitute; stir 1 minute. Simmer 2 minutes.

Ladle 1 cup of soup into a bowl, and top with chopped green onions. Serve immediately.

MAKES 4 SERVINGS
SERVING SIZE: 1 CUP
CALORIES: 148 • CHOL.: 0 • FAT: 5 G. • SODIUM: 374 MG.

Seafood Chowder

This kind of dish was the origin of bouillabaisse. This version is thickened with puréed vegetables instead of cream. Serve this treat to yourself or the family. Freeze leftovers.

Prepare Ahead

Onion**

1 Tbsp. MARGARINE

1 cup chopped ONIONS** or sliced LEEKS

1 cup chopped CARROTS

1 cup chopped CELERY

3 cups peeled, diced POTATOES

1 BAY LEAF

1/2 tsp. SALT

1/2 tsp. dried THYME

1 can (10 oz.) chopped CLAMS, drained, liquid reserved

1 lb. FLOUNDER or HALIBUT, cut in 2-inch pieces

2 cups LOW-FAT MILK

1/2 tsp. HOT PEPPER SAUCE

In 3-quart saucepan heat margarine over medium heat. Add onions, carrots, and celery; sauté 3 minutes. Stir in potatoes, bay leaf, salt, and thyme. Combine reserved liquid from clams and enough water to equal 3/4 cup; add to saucepan. Simmer 15 minutes or until vegetables are tender. Purée half the chowder mixture and return to saucepan. Add fish; simmer 5 to 8 minutes or just until cooked. Stir in milk and clams. Heat through. (Do not boil.) Stir in hot pepper sauce. Remove bay leaf before serving.

MAKES 8 CUPS

SERVING SIZE: 1 CUP

CALORIES: 160 • CHOL.: 35 MG. • FAT: 3 G. • SODIUM: 390 MG.

Zucchini Soup

Quick and Easy

Onion**

1-1/2 cups ZUCCHINI, sliced, plus 4 paper-thin slices
3 leaves of fresh BASIL, chopped, or 1/2 tsp. dried basil
1/2 cup chopped ONION**
1/2 cup CELERY
1/2 cup low-sodium CHICKEN BROTH
SALT and PEPPER to taste

Put all ingredients in a pot and simmer for 30 minutes. Put in blender and blend. Serve hot with slices of raw zucchini on top for garnish.

MAKES 2 SERVINGS
SERVING SIZE: 1 CUP
CALORIES: 40 • CHOL.: 0 • FAT: 0 • SODIUM: 253 MG.

Zucchini Soup with Curry

Quick and Easy • Prepare Ahead

2 Tbsp. OIL
4 medium ZUCCHINI, cut in 1-inch cubes
1/2 cup sliced GREEN ONIONS**
1-1/2 tsp. CURRY POWDER*
1 can (13 oz.) CHICKEN BROTH
1 Tbsp. CORNSTARCH
1/2 cup APPLE JUICE
1 cup PLAIN NONFAT YOGURT**
1/8 tsp. PEPPER

In large saucepan heat oil over medium heat. Add zucchini, green onions, and curry powder; sauté 5 minutes or until onions are tender. Add broth; reduce heat. Cover and simmer 30 minutes or until zucchini is tender. In small bowl mix cornstarch and apple juice until smooth; whisk into soup. Over medium heat, bring soup to a boil and boil 1 minute. Pour into blender or food processor; add yogurt and pepper. Blend or process until smooth. Serve hot or chilled. If reheated, do not boil!

MAKES 4 SERVINGS
SERVING SIZE: 1 CUP
CALORIES: 170 • CHOL.: 5 MG. • FAT: 9 G. • SODIUM: 580 MG.

Broccoli Pasta Salad

Quick and Easy • Prepare Ahead

Mayonnaise*, Onion**, Lemon peel & Juice**

3/4 cup REDUCED-CALORIE MAYONNAISE* (check label)

1/4 cup sliced GREEN ONIONS**

1/4 cup SKIM MILK

2 Tbsp. chopped PARSLEY

2 tsp. LEMON JUICE**

1 tsp. grated LEMON PEEL**

1-1/2 cups (4 oz.) PASTA RUFFLES, cooked and drained

1 cup cooked (approx. 3 minutes) BROCCOLI FLORETS

1/2 cup cooked sliced CARROTS

In large bowl stir mayonnaise, green onion, skim milk, parsley, lemon juice, and lemon peel until smooth. Add cooked pasta ruffles, broccoli, and carrots; toss to coat well. Cover, and chill for 2 to 6 hours before serving.

MAKES 4 SERVINGS

SERVING SIZE: 1 CUP

CALORIES: 140 • CHOL.: 0 • FAT: 5 G. • SODIUM: 130 MG.

Crunchy 3-Bean Salad

Quick and Easy • Prepare Ahead

Beans*

I can (15 oz.) KIDNEY BEANS*
I can (15 oz.) FRENCH-STYLE GREEN BEANS*, drained
I can (15 oz.) GARBANZO BEANS*
10 PEPPERONCINI PEPPERS, sliced
I jar (20 oz.) PIMENTO
3/4 cup mild WHITE VINEGAR
2 Tbsp. OLIVE OIL
I tsp. GROUND OREGANO
I Tbsp. sodium-free SALT SUBSTITUTE

Combine beans, peppers, and pimento in mixing bowl. Mix remaining ingredients together in separate bowl. Pour dressing over bean mixture. Marinate 1 hour in refrigerator.

MAKES 6 SERVINGS
SERVING SIZE: I CUP
CALORIES: 215 • CHOL.: 0 • FAT: 6 G. • SODIUM: 154 MG.

Chunky Tomato-Mushroom Salad

Quick and Easy

Mushrooms*, Walnuts**

2 cups TOMATO chunks (about 3/4 lb.)
1 cup sliced fresh MUSHROOMS*
1 Tbsp. chopped WALNUTS**
1 Tbsp. chopped fresh BASIL
1 Tbsp. WATER
1 Tbsp. WHITE VINEGAR
1/8 tsp. SALT
2 tsp. VEGETABLE OIL

Combine tomato chunks, mushrooms, and walnuts in a bowl; toss gently. Combine basil, water, vinegar, salt, and vegetable oil in a jar; cover tightly and shake vigorously. Pour over tomato mixture, and toss gently.

MAKES 6 SERVINGS
SERVING SIZE: 1/2 CUP
CALORIES: 37 • CHOL.: 0 • FAT: 2.4 G. • SODIUM: 54 MG.

Chicken-Vegetable Salad

Quick and Easy

Mayonnaise*, Onion**

2 cups chopped CHICKEN BREAST
1/2 CUCUMBER, peeled and diced
1/2 cup diced CELERY
1/4 cup diced GREEN PEPPER
1/4 cup chopped PIMENTO
1/2 cup drained and sliced WATER CHESTNUTS
2 Tbsp. sliced SCALLIONS**
1/4 cup MAYONNAISE* (check label)
SALAD GREENS
2 Tbsp. CAPERS
PAPRIKA

Toss chicken, cucumber, celery, green pepper, pimento, water chestnuts, and scallions with mayonnaise. Serve on crisp salad greens, garnished with capers and paprika.

MAKES 6 SERVINGS
SERVING SIZE: 3/4 CUP
CALORIES: 153 • CHOL.: 40.5 MG. • FAT: 8.8 G. • SODIUM: 97.7 MG.

Couscous & Vegetable Salad

High in vitamin C, this winner can easily
be prepared in advance to marry the flavors.

Prepare Ahead

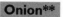

I cup uncooked COUSCOUS

1/4 cup VEGETABLE OIL

2 Tbsp. WHITE VINEGAR

3 Tbsp. chopped FRESH BASIL or 3 Tbsp. chopped PARSLEY plus I tsp. dried BASIL

I small CLOVE GARLIC, minced or pressed

I tsp. SALT

1/4 tsp. PEPPER

2 medium TOMATOES, diced

I small ZUCCHINI, cut in matchstick strips

I small RED or GREEN PEPPER, cut in matchstick strips

4 GREEN ONIONS**, thinly sliced

2 Tbsp. sliced pitted ripe OLIVES

Prepare couscous according to package directions; cool. In large bowl combine oil, vinegar, basil, garlic, salt, and pepper. Add couscous, tomatoes, zucchini, red pepper, green onions, and olives; toss to coat well. Cover, and chill.

MAKES 8 SERVINGS

SERVING SIZE: I CUP

CALORIES: 90 • CHOL.: 0 • FAT: 8 G. • SODIUM: 370 MG.

Cuke Salad

Quick and Easy • Prepare Ahead

Mayonnaise*, Onion**, Walnuts**

1 pkg. SUGAR-FREE LIME GELATIN
1/2 cup boiling WATER
1 Tbsp. WHITE VINEGAR
1/2 cup chopped WALNUTS**
1/2 cup chopped CELERY
1/2 cup LOW-FAT MAYONNAISE* (check label)
1 small ONION**, chopped
1 medium CUCUMBER, diced
1 lb. LOW-FAT COTTAGE CHEESE
1 can (8 oz.) unsweetened PINEAPPLE BITS, including juice

Dissolve gelatin in hot water. Add vinegar and remaining ingredients. Chill in refrigerator until firm.

MAKES 8 SERVINGS
SERVING SIZE: 3/4 CUP
CALORIES: 180 • CHOL.: 3 MG. • FAT: 11 G. • SODIUM: 232 MG.

Harlequin Slaw

This dish is just right for a picnic, no matter what the season.

Quick and Easy • *Prepare Ahead*

Salad dressing*, Onion**, Lemon juice**

3 cups coarsely shredded RED CABBAGE

1/2 cup drained, canned, no-salt-added WHOLE KERNEL CORN

2 Tbsp. minced fresh PARSLEY

2 tsp. LEMON JUICE**

2 Tbsp. chopped GREEN ONIONS**

1/4 cup diced GREEN BELL PEPPER

3 Tbsp. LOW-CALORIE SLAW DRESSING* (check label)

Combine all ingredients in a bowl; toss well.

MAKES 8 SERVINGS

SERVING SIZE: 1/2 CUP

CALORIES: 36 • CHOL.: 4 MG. • FAT: 1.3 G. • SODIUM: 15 MG.

Garden Fresh Tuna Salad

A colorful, flavorful combination of vegetables to add to an ordinary tuna salad dish. Minced garlic is available in small glass jars for convenience; find it in the produce department, and keep in the refrigerator.

Quick and Easy • Prepare Ahead

Mayonnaise*, Onion**

2/3 cup REDUCED-CALORIE MAYONNAISE* (check label)

2 Tbsp. DIJON MUSTARD

2 Tbsp. SKIM MILK

I CLOVE GARLIC, minced

I lb. small NEW POTATOES, halved, cooked, and cooled

2 cans (6-1/2 oz. each) WATER-PACKED TUNA, drained

I YELLOW, RED, or GREEN PEPPER, cut in strips

1-1/2 cups fresh GREEN BEANS, cut and cooked,
    or I pkg. (16 oz.) frozen CUT GREEN BEANS, thawed

1-1/2 cups halved CHERRY TOMATOES

1/4 cup minced RED ONION**

LETTUCE

In large bowl combine mayonnaise, mustard, milk, and garlic. Add potatoes, tuna, pepper, green beans, tomatoes, and onion; toss to coat. Cover; chill. Serve on a bed of lettuce.

MAKES 8 SERVINGS

SERVING SIZE: I CUP

CALORIES: 210 • CHOL.: 10 MG. • FAT: 7 G. • SODIUM: 340 MG.

Garden Pasta Salad

The yellow squash, cherry tomatoes, and green peppers
help dress up this carbo-rich salad without unwanted calories.

Quick and Easy

Mayonnaise*

3/4 cup REDUCED-CALORIE MAYONNAISE* (check label)
1/2 cup fresh PARSLEY LEAVES
2 Tbsp. WHITE VINEGAR
1 tsp. DRIED BASIL
1 CLOVE GARLIC
1-1/2 cups (4 oz.) MACARONI TWISTS, cooked and drained
2 cups sliced YELLOW SQUASH
1-1/2 cups CHERRY TOMATOES, quartered
1 cup diced GREEN PEPPER
LETTUCE

In blender or food processor combine mayonnaise, parsley, vinegar, basil and garlic; blend or process until smooth. In large bowl combine macaroni, squash, tomatoes, and green pepper. Add dressing; toss to coat well. Serve on lettuce-lined platter.

MAKES 6 SERVINGS
SERVING SIZE: 1 CUP
CALORIES: 190 • CHOL.: 0 • FAT: 6 G. • SODIUM: 160 MG.

Green Grape & Apple Waldorf Salad

An old-time favorite variation (first made by the chef at the Waldorf-Astoria Hotel in the 1890s) that has been revived for the 1990s. Serve with meatloaf and Brussel sprouts. Preparation time: 13 minutes.

Quick and Easy

Mayonnaise*, Pecans**, Yogurt**

1 cup chopped RED APPLE
1/2 cup GREEN GRAPES
1/4 cup chopped CELERY
1 Tbsp. chopped PECANS**
1 Tbsp. unsweetened APPLE JUICE
1 Tbsp. PLAIN NONFAT YOGURT**
1 Tbsp. REDUCED-CALORIE MAYONNAISE*
4 LETTUCE LEAVES

Combine apple, grapes, celery, and pecans in a bowl; toss gently. Combine apple juice, yogurt, and mayonnaise in a bowl, stirring with a wire whisk until smooth. Pour over apple mixture; toss well. Serve on lettuce-lined salad plates.

MAKES 4 SERVINGS
SERVING SIZE: 1/2 CUP
CALORIES: 60 • CHOL.: 1 MG. • FAT: 2.5 G. • SODIUM: 39 MG.

Jicama Salad

Quick and Easy • Prepare Ahead

Green onions**, Yogurt**, Sour cream**

2 pkgs. (10 oz. each) frozen tiny GREEN PEAS, thawed
3 cups BEAN SPROUTS, fresh or canned
1 JICAMA, peeled and chopped into 1-1/2 inch pieces
1 cup chopped CELERY
1 bunch GREEN ONIONS**, chopped
1 cup PLAIN NONFAT YOGURT**
1 Tbsp. REDUCED-FAT SOUR CREAM**
PEPPER to taste

Drain peas well. Combine peas, bean sprouts, jicama, celery, and green onions. Combine yogurt, sour cream, and pepper; toss with vegetables. Refrigerate until ready to serve.

MAKES 6 SERVINGS
SERVING SIZE: 1-1/4 CUPS
CALORIES: 152 • CHOL.: 1 MG. • FAT: 3 G. • SODIUM: 161 MG.

Mandarin Salad

Quick and Easy • Prepare Ahead

Mandarin oranges**, Onion**

2 cups HEAD LETTUCE, torn in pieces
2 cups ROMAINE LETTUCE, torn in pieces
1 cup chopped CELERY
1 GREEN ONION**, chopped
1/2 tsp. SALT
dash PEPPER
1 Tbsp. SUGAR
2 Tbsp. WHITE VINEGAR
1 Tbsp. OLIVE OIL
dash TABASCO SAUCE
1 can (10-11 oz.) MANDARIN ORANGES**, chilled

Toss lettuce, celery, and onion. In a separate bowl, combine salt, pepper, sugar, vinegar, olive oil, and Tabasco sauce to make dressing. Drizzle 2 teaspoons dressing on lettuce. Top with mandarin oranges.

Salad and dressing can be prepared separately ahead of time and refrigerated until ready to serve.

MAKES 6 SERVINGS
SERVING SIZE: 3/4 CUP
CALORIES: 89 • CHOL.: 0 • FAT: 5 G. • SODIUM: 4 MG.

Strawberry-Banana Salad

Be sure the banana is not overripe, as the tyramine content,
a blood pressure agent, increases with ripeness.

Quick and Easy • Prepare Ahead

Yogurt**, Banana**

1 pkg. (3 oz.) SUGAR-FREE STRAWBERRY GELATIN
1 envelope (.25 oz.) UNFLAVORED GELATIN
1-1/4 cups boiling WATER
1 cup fresh or unsweetened frozen WHOLE STRAWBERRIES
1/2 cup LOW-FAT COTTAGE CHEESE
1/2 cup LOW-FAT STRAWBERRY-BANANA YOGURT**
1 large BANANA** (not too ripe), cut into 1 inch chunks

Place strawberry gelatin and unflavored gelatin in a blender. Turn blender on low speed and slowly add boiling water. Blend until gelatins are dissolved. Turn blender up to medium speed and slowly add strawberries. Blend until smooth. Turn off blender and add remaining ingredients. Blend on medium speed until smooth and no cottage cheese particles can be seen.

Pour mixture into a 9-inch square pan. Refrigerate for 2 hours before serving. Cut into squares to serve.

NOTE: This recipe can be doubled and put into a mold. To serve as a dessert, pour the mixture into a graham cracker crumb pie crust and chill.

MAKES 9 SERVINGS
SERVING SIZE: 1/2 CUP
CALORIES: 40 • CHOL.: 1 MG. • FAT: 0.5 G. • SODIUM: 88 MG.

Taco Salad

Fill preformed taco shells or, if you prefer the tortilla wedges, bake and serve separately. Add a tall, cool beverage for a complete meal.

Easy

NONSTICK COOKING SPRAY

1 pkg. (12 pieces) CORN TORTILLAS cut into wedges, or preformed and cooked TACO SALAD SHELLS

1-1/4 lbs. EXTRA LEAN GROUND BEEF

1 jar (8-oz.) CHUNKY SALSA

1 can (8-3/4 oz.) PINTO BEANS**, drained and rinsed

1 HEAD LETTUCE, washed, dried, and torn

2 TOMATOES, cut into wedges

1 CUCUMBER, peeled and diced

1 GREEN PEPPER, seeded and chopped

2 GREEN ONIONS**, diced, tops included

8 BLACK OLIVES (optional)

Preheat oven to 350 degrees. Place tortillas on 2 baking sheets sprayed with cooking spray. Sprinkle with salt, if desired, and bake 12 minutes. Turn them over and continue baking for an additional 5 minutes.

Brown meat in skillet or microwave oven. Drain well. Mix meat with 1 cup salsa and the pinto beans. Refrigerate.

Combine lettuce, tomato, cucumber, green pepper, and green onion in bowl. Refrigerate. When ready to serve, combine lettuce mixture and meat mixture. Garnish with black olives, if desired. Serve with tortilla chips prepared as above or fill taco salad shells. Use additional salsa as dressing.

MAKES 6 SERVINGS
SERVING SIZE: 1 CUP OF SALAD MIXTURE, 2 CORN TORTILLAS
CALORIES: 397 • CHOL.: 67 MG. • FAT: 13 G. • SODIUM: 247 MG.

Tuna and Brown Rice Salad

Substitute bulgur for the brown rice if you like. The rice (or bulgur) and peas have the right combination of amino acids to make a complete protein. There's plenty of that here!

Easy • Prepare Ahead

Lemon juice**, Sour cream**

1-1/4 cups (1/2 cup dry) cooked BROWN RICE
1 can (6-1/2 oz.) TUNA IN WATER, drained
1 pkg. (10 oz.) frozen PEAS, thawed
1/2 cup LOW-FAT SOUR CREAM**
1/2 cup shredded CARROT
1 tsp. PREPARED MUSTARD
1-1/2 tsp. LEMON JUICE**
1/8 tsp. PEPPER
pinch SALT
LETTUCE LEAVES
16 UNSALTED CRACKERS

Mix together the rice, tuna, peas, sour cream, carrot, mustard, lemon juice, pepper, and salt in a large bowl.

Arrange lettuce leaves on 4 plates. Using ice cream scoop, scoop about 1 cup tuna mixture on each plate of lettuce. Serve with 4 crackers each.

MAKES 4 SERVINGS
SERVING SIZE: 1 CUP
CALORIES: 346 • CHOL.: 26 MG. • FAT: 7 G. • SODIUM: 451 MG.

---

*=Dangerous to some • **=Consume with caution • See pages 19-22 for more information

Tuna Pasta Salad à la Niçoise

A pasta variation for tuna salad; the red onions
and green beans add color and crunch.

Easy • Prepare Ahead

Mayonnaise*, Onion**, Lime peel**, Lime juice**

1 cup REDUCED-CALORIE MAYONNAISE* (check label)

2 Tbsp. LIME JUICE**

1 tsp. grated LIME PEEL**

1/2 tsp. DRIED TARRAGON

2 cups (4-1/2 oz. dry) SEA SHELL MACARONI, cooked and drained

1 pkg. (9 oz.) frozen GREEN BEANS, cooked, drained, and chilled

1 can (6-1/2 oz.) WATER-PACKED TUNA, drained and flaked

1/2 cup coarsely chopped RED ONION**

6 LETTUCE LEAVES

TOMATOES for garnish

In large bowl stir mayonnaise, lime juice, grated lime peel, and tarragon until smooth. Add macaroni, green beans, tuna, and onion. Cover; chill at least 2 hours to blend flavors. Arrange on lettuce-lined platter. Garnish with tomatoes and serve with a cup of hot Creamy Romano Tomato Soup (see Soups).

MAKES 6 SERVINGS

SERVING SIZE: 1 CUP

CALORIES: 250 • CHOL.: 5 MG. • FAT: 9 G. • SODIUM: 290 MG.

Spanish Potato Salad

A hot potato salad that can be made ahead of time and reheated for a party, where it will be a favorite with everyone. Always taste before serving and adjust seasonings.

Easy

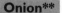

1/4 cup MARGARINE
1/4 cup WHITE VINEGAR
1 Tbsp. SUGAR
1/4 tsp. PEPPER
1/4 tsp. DRY MUSTARD
1/3 cup finely chopped GREEN PEPPER
1/3 cup finely chopped ONION**
1/4 cup diced PIMENTOS
8 medium POTATOES, peeled, diced, and cooked.

Melt margarine and combine with vinegar, sugar, pepper, and dry mustard. Mix in green pepper, onion, and pimento. Pour over drained warm potatoes and serve immediately.

MAKES 10 SERVINGS
SERVING SIZE: 3/4 CUP
CALORIES: 103 • CHOL.: 0 • FAT: 5.G. • SODIUM: 43 MG.

Catalina Salad Dressing

*A make-ahead, low-calorie dressing for mixed greens or salads
or a zesty addition for lean cuts of meat and poultry.*

Easy • Prepare Ahead

Lemon juice**, Onion**

- 3-1/2 cups (28 oz. can) crushed TOMATOES
- 1/2 cup finely chopped GREEN PEPPER
- 1/3 cup sliced SHALLOTS**
- 1/3 cup WHITE VINEGAR
- 1/4 cup finely chopped PARSLEY
- 3 Tbsp. fresh LEMON JUICE**
- 1 tsp. dried OREGANO LEAVES, crushed
- 1 tsp. GARLIC SALT
- 1/2 tsp. DRIED TARRAGON LEAVES, crushed
- 1/2 tsp. DRY MUSTARD
- 1/4 tsp. BLACK PEPPER

Combine all ingredients in a large bowl. Cover, and refrigerate for 3 to
4 hours to allow flavors to blend. Serve over salad greens.

MAKES 4 CUPS
SERVING SIZE: 2 TABLESPOONS
CALORIES: 18 • CHOL.: 0 • FAT: 0 • SODIUM: 260 MG.

---

*=Dangerous to some • **=Consume with caution • See pages 19-22 for more information

Creamy (Blender) Mayonnaise

Homemade mayonnaise has an appeal over commercial because you have control over the ingredients! If your mayonnaise starts to separate, add more of the combining agent, egg.

Quick and Easy

Onion powder**

1/3 cup EGG SUBSTITUTE
1 tsp. DRY MUSTARD
1/2 tsp. PAPRIKA
2 Tbsp. WHITE VINEGAR
1/4 tsp. ONION POWDER**
dash GROUND RED PEPPER
1 cup VEGETABLE OIL

Combine the first six ingredients with 1/2 cup oil in a blender container. Cover and blend on medium-high speed just until mixed. Without turning blender off, very slowly pour in other 1/2 cup oil in a fine steady stream. If necessary, use rubber spatula to keep mixture flowing to blades. Continue blending until oil is completely incorporated and mixture is smooth and thick. Store in refrigerator.

MAKES 1-1/2 CUPS
SERVING SIZE: 1 TABLESPOON
CALORIES: 45 • CHOL.: 0 • FAT: 5 G. • SODIUM: 4 MG.

---

*=Dangerous to some • **=Consume with caution • See pages 19-22 for more information

Basic Italian Dressing

Quick and Easy • Prepare Ahead

---

    1 cup VEGETABLE OIL
    1 cup WHITE VINEGAR
    2 tsp. SUGAR
    DRY MUSTARD
    BASIL LEAVES
    TARRAGON LEAVES
    DILL WEED or OREGANO LEAVES

Combine oil, vinegar, and sugar in jar with tight-fitting lid and shake vigorously. Season to taste with dry mustard, basil, tarragon, dill, or oregano. Store in refrigerator.

MAKES 1-1/2 CUPS
SERVING SIZE: 1 TABLESPOON
CALORIES: 82 • CHOL.: 0 • FAT: 9 G. • SODIUM: 0

Cucumber Dressing

This can be used as a substitute for tartar sauce with fish or on baked potatoes for a reduced-calorie topping.

Quick and Easy

Lemon juice**, Onion**

1 cup 1% LOW-FAT COTTAGE CHEESE
1/4 cup SKIM MILK
2 Tbsp. chopped fresh PARSLEY
2 Tbsp. sliced GREEN ONIONS**
1 Tbsp. LEMON JUICE**
1-1/2 tsp. PREPARED HORSERADISH
1/2 cup seeded, diced, CUCUMBER

Combine cottage cheese, skim milk, parsley, onions, lemon juice, and horseradish in an electric blender; cover and process until smooth. Add cucumber, and process just until coarsely chopped. Serve over lettuce wedges.

MAKES 1-3/4 CUPS
SERVING SIZE: 1 TABLESPOON
CALORIES: 7 • CHOL.: 0 • FAT: 0.1 G. • SODIUM: 34 MG.

Sprout Dressing

If you want some variety in your salads, try preparing this healthy and tasty dressing.

Quick and Easy

Lemon juice**

1-1/2 cups ALFALFA or RADISH SPROUTS
1/2 cup VEGETABLE OIL
2 Tbsp. LEMON JUICE** or WHITE VINEGAR
1/2 tsp. PREPARED MUSTARD
SALT and PEPPER to taste

Combine all ingredients in blender. Blend until smooth, about 1 minute. Serve on salad or use as fruit or vegetable dip. Store in refrigerator.

MAKES 2 CUPS
SERVING SIZE: 1 TABLESPOON
CALORIES: 86 • CHOL.: 0 • FAT: 9 G. • SODIUM: 1 MG.

Egg Salad Dressing

The eggs add a satisfying but low-calorie richness to this dressing.

Quick and Easy

Lemon juice**

3 hard-cooked EGGS or 3/4 cup EGG SUBSTITUTE, cooked
2 Tbsp. WATER
1 Tbsp. WHITE VINEGAR
2 tsp. LEMON JUICE**
SALT and PEPPER to taste
GARLIC POWDER to taste

Put eggs in blender and blend. Add water, vinegar, and lemon juice. Add salt, pepper, and garlic powder to taste. Blend until mixture is creamy.

MAKES 1/2 CUP
SERVING SIZE: 1 TABLESPOON
CALORIES: 41 • CHOL.: 137 MG. • FAT: 3 G. • SODIUM: 35 MG.

---

*=Dangerous to some • **=Consume with caution • See pages 19-22 for more information

Flavorful French Dressing

This quickly assembled salad dressing is a great favorite with everyone.
Tasty with both vegetable and fruit salads.

Quick and Easy

Onion**

1/2 cup VEGETABLE OIL
1/2 cup WHITE VINEGAR
1 tsp. SALT
1 Tbsp. grated ONION**, or 1 Tbsp. minced
DEHYDRATED ONION**
1/2 cup SUGAR
1/4 cup KETCHUP
1 tsp. PAPRIKA

Combine all ingredients in large jar (you may prefer to make a half recipe). Shake well before serving. Store in refrigerator.

MAKES APPROXIMATELY 1 PINT
SERVING SIZE: 1 TABLESPOON
CALORIES: 67 • CHOL.: 0 • FAT: 6.4 G. • SODIUM: 214 MG.

Vegetable Entrées

Cajun Rice

Quick and Easy

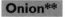

2 Tbsp. OIL
1 cup uncooked REGULAR RICE
1 large ONION**, chopped
1 large GREEN PEPPER, chopped
1 Tbsp. minced GARLIC
1 can (14-1/2 oz.) STEWED TOMATOES, undrained
1-1/4 cups WATER
1/2 tsp. HOT PEPPER SAUCE

In medium skillet, heat oil over medium-high heat. Stir in rice, onion, pepper, and garlic. Sauté 3 minutes. Stir in tomatoes, water, and hot pepper sauce, breaking tomatoes with a spoon. Bring to a boil, then reduce heat. Cover and simmer 20 minutes, stirring occasionally, or until liquid is absorbed and rice is tender.

MAKES 8 SERVINGS
SERVING SIZE: 3/4 CUP
CALORIES: 140 • CHOL.: 0 • FAT: 4 G. • SODIUM: 135 MG.

Linguine with Tomato Sauce

Quick and Easy

2 Tbsp. VEGETABLE OIL

3 CLOVES GARLIC, minced or pressed

1-1/2 lbs. ripe ROMANO TOMATOES, coarsely chopped

2 cups loosely packed, chopped fresh BASIL,
    or 2 cups chopped PARSLEY plus 1 Tbsp. dried BASIL

2 Tbsp. WHITE VINEGAR

8 oz. LINGUINE, cooked and drained

In large skillet heat oil over medium-high heat. Add garlic; sauté 1 minute. Stir in tomatoes; bring to boil. Reduce heat, cover, and simmer 5 minutes, stirring occasionally, or until sauce thickens slightly. Stir in basil and vinegar. Serve with linguine.

MAKES 4 SERVINGS

SERVING SIZE: 2/3 CUP

CALORIES: 320 • CHOL.: 0 • FAT: 8 G. • SODIUM: 25 MG.

Carrot-Broccoli-Mushroom Stir-Fry

Stir-fry originated because of the Oriental shortage of fuels. The result was many small, quickly cooked, but not overly cooked, ingredients.

Quick and Easy

Mushroom*, Onion**, Lemon juice**

1 lb. fresh BROCCOLI
1 Tbsp. MARGARINE
1 Tbsp. VEGETABLE OIL
1 lb. CARROTS, peeled and thinly sliced
3/4 lb. MUSHROOMS*, sliced thin
3 medium GREEN ONIONS**
1 tsp. LEMON JUICE**
2 Tbsp. WHITE VINEGAR
1 tsp. NUTMEG
1 tsp. THYME
PEPPER to taste

Wash broccoli. Peel stems and cut into 1-inch lengths. Separate broccoli florets by cutting into quarters so they are of uniform size.

In a large skillet or wok, heat margarine and oil over medium heat. Add broccoli, carrots, mushrooms and onions. Cook and stir until vegetables are tender-crisp, about 5 minutes. Stir in remaining ingredients, and serve immediately.

MAKES 8 SERVINGS
SERVING SIZE: 2/3 CUP
CALORIES: 93 • CHOL.: 0 • FAT: 3.7 G. • SODIUM: 61.6 MG

Green Bean & Rice Casserole

A casserole that is easy to make and is an economical taste treat. The beans and rice combination serves as a complete protein replacement for meat.

Prepare Ahead

Mushrooms*, Onion**

1 can (10-3/4 oz.) condensed CREAM OF MUSHROOM SOUP*
1/2 cup SKIM MILK
1/2 tsp. DRIED MARJORAM
1/4 tsp. GARLIC POWDER
1/8 tsp. PEPPER
1 pkg. (9 oz.) frozen FRENCH-STYLE GREEN BEANS, cooked and drained
1/4 cup sliced GREEN ONIONS**
3 cups COOKED RICE, unsalted
PAPRIKA

Preheat oven to 350 degrees. In 1-1/2 quart casserole, combine soup, milk, marjoram, garlic powder, and pepper. Stir in beans, green onions and rice. Cover, and bake for 25 minutes or until hot and bubbling. Sprinkle with paprika. Bake uncovered 5 minutes more.

MICROWAVE: In large bowl, combine soup, milk, marjoram, garlic powder, and pepper. Stir in beans, green onions, and rice. Spread rice mixture evenly in a 12 x 8-inch microwave-proof baking dish. Cover with vented plastic wrap; microwave on high (100% power) 10 minutes or until edges are bubbling and center is hot, rotating dish once halfway through heating. Sprinkle with paprika. Microwave uncovered 1 minute.

TIP: To reduce sodium content, use low-sodium soup.

MAKES 6 SERVINGS
SERVING SIZE: 2/3 CUP
CALORIES: 218 • CHOL.: 5 MG. • FAT: 7 G. • SODIUM: 562 MG.

*=Dangerous to some • **=Consume with caution • See pages 19-22 for more information

Mediterranean Vegetables

This Middle Eastern entrée features eggplant, so popular in that part of the world. Add the touch of thyme for pizzazz.

Easy

Onion**

1 Tbsp. MARGARINE
1-1/2 cups sliced ONIONS**
1 cup GREEN PEPPER strips
1/2 tsp. crushed fresh GARLIC
1 can (16 oz.) LOW-SODIUM TOMATOES, coarsely chopped
2 cups cubed unpeeled EGGPLANT
1-1/2 cups thickly sliced ZUCCHINI
1/4 tsp. THYME leaves
1 BAY LEAF
dash PEPPER

Melt margarine in a large heavy pan over medium heat. Add onions, green pepper, and garlic. Sauté, stirring occasionally, until onions are transparent, about 5 minutes. Mix in tomatoes, eggplant, zucchini, thyme, bay leaf, and pepper. Cover and simmer over medium-low heat, stirring occasionally, until vegetables are tender, about 15 minutes. Remove cover and cook an additional 5 to 10 minutes. Remove bay leaf.

MICROWAVE: In 3-quart microwave-safe casserole, combine all ingredients except tomatoes. Cover, microwave on high (100% power) for 8 minutes. Stir in tomatoes. Cover, and microwave on high for 5 to 7 minutes.

MAKES 4 SERVINGS
SERVING SIZE: 1-1/2 CUPS
CALORIES: 93 • CHOL.: 0 • FAT: 3 G. • SODIUM: 44 MG.

Mexicali Rice

Spanish rice didn't become famous for nothing.
Make this as hot as you like with the hot pepper sauce.

Prepare Ahead

Onion**

2 Tbsp. MARGARINE
1/2 cup chopped ONION**
1/4 cup chopped GREEN PEPPER
1/4 tsp. crushed fresh GARLIC
1 cup uncooked LONG GRAIN RICE
2-1/4 cups WATER
1/2 cup (4 cubes) frozen LOW-SODIUM TOMATO BASE,
    or TOMATO FRESH SALSA (see Sauces)
1/4 tsp. OREGANO LEAVES
1/8 tsp. BLACK PEPPER
3-4 drops HOT PEPPER SAUCE

In large skillet, melt margarine over medium heat. Stir in onion, green pepper, and garlic; sauté until tender, stirring occasionally, 2 to 2-1/2 minutes. Stir in rice; cook and stir until golden, about 1-1/2 to 2 minutes. Add water, tomato base, oregano, pepper, and hot pepper sauce. Cook and stir until tomato base melts. Reduce heat to low; cover and cook until rice is tender and liquid is absorbed, 20 to 25 minutes. Fluff rice with fork and serve hot.

MICROWAVE: In a 2-quart microwave-safe casserole, melt margarine on high (100% power) for 40 to 45 seconds. Add onion, green pepper, and garlic; microwave on high for 2 minutes, stirring after 1 minute. Stir in rice, water, tomato base, oregano, pepper, and hot pepper sauce. Cover; microwave on high for 18 to 20 minutes, stirring after 9 minutes. Let stand 2 to 3 minutes; stir before serving.

MAKES 6 SERVINGS
SERVING SIZE: 2/3 CUP
CALORIES: 167 • CHOL.: 0 • FAT: 4 G. • SODIUM: 41 MG.

Ratatouille

Simple proof that lack of fat need not compromise flavor. Eggplant easily picks up the flavor of the other ingredients. Serve with rice and very lean ground beef.

Prepare Ahead

Onion**

I small GREEN PEPPER
I medium ONION**
I tsp. VEGETABLE OIL
I medium TOMATO
I medium ZUCCHINI (I/2 lb.)
I small EGGPLANT (3/4 lb.)
I GARLIC CLOVE, minced
I/2 tsp. DRIED BASIL
I/2 tsp. DRIED THYME
2 Tbsp. minced fresh PARSLEY leaves

Cut the green pepper into strips. Slice the onion. Sauté pepper and onion in oil. Chop the tomato, and slice the zucchini into 1/4-inch-thick slices. Cube the eggplant. Add the tomato, zucchini, eggplant, garlic, basil, thyme, and parsley to the pepper and onion mixture. Simmer until the vegetables are tender.

MAKES 4 SERVINGS
SERVING SIZE: 3/4 CUP
CALORIES: 47 • CHOL.: 0 • FAT: 2 G. • SODIUM: 7 MG.

Red Chile Linguine

The traditional linguine comes with more than its share of saturated fat.

Prepare Ahead

Lime juice**

1/4 cup OLIVE OIL
2 tsp. GARLIC, minced
1/2 tsp. RED PEPPER FLAKES
8 oz. LINGUINE, cooked
1/4 cup PARSLEY, chopped
1 LIME**, juiced

Heat olive oil in skillet; add garlic, and sauté 1 minute. Add red pepper, and sauté 30 seconds. Add cooked linguine; stir well and cook over medium heat until hot and well coated. Add parsley, and stir well; add lime juice. Toss well and serve.

MAKES 6 SERVINGS
SERVING SIZE: 2/3 CUP
CALORIES: 364 • CHOL.: 0 • FAT: 10 G. • SODIUM: 8 MG.

Rice-Stuffed Squash

Very flavorful because of the contrast of crunchy walnuts, squash, and orange.

Easy

Orange rind**, Orange juice**, Walnuts**

2 medium ACORN SQUASH
1/2 cup (dry) RICE, cooked
1/2 cup chopped WALNUTS**
1 tsp. grated ORANGE RIND**
1-2 Tbsp. frozen ORANGE JUICE CONCENTRATE**

Preheat oven to 400 degrees. Cut the squash in half and remove the seeds. Combine the remaining ingredients and fill the squash with the mixture. Place in a baking pan; cover with aluminum foil or lid and bake for about 35 minutes or until squash is fork-tender. Extra orange juice concentrate can be drizzled over the squash just before serving, if desired.

MAKES 4 SERVINGS
SERVING SIZE: 1/2 SQUASH
CALORIES: 204 • CHOL.: 0 • FAT: 10 G. • SODIUM: 20 MG.

Spaghetti Squash 'n Sauce

An inexpensive main dish, easy to fix and colorful, for spaghetti squash devotees. Increase the cottage cheese on the side for protein.

Quick and Easy

1 YELLOW SPAGHETTI SQUASH
1 jar (32 oz.) SPAGHETTI SAUCE
4 tsp. COTTAGE CHEESE

Preheat oven to 350 degrees. Poke spaghetti squash several times with long fork. Place on baking sheet. Bake for 1 hour. Cut squash in half and remove seeds. Pull spaghetti strands free with a fork. Heat spaghetti sauce. For each serving, ladle 1 cup sauce onto 1 cup spaghetti squash. Top with 1 teaspoon cottage cheese.

MICROWAVE: Poke spaghetti squash several times with long fork. Place in microwave-safe baking dish. Microwave on high (100% power) 4 to 6 minutes. Turn squash over and microwave for another 4 to 6 minutes. Remove from oven and let stand 5 to 10 minutes. Cut squash in half and remove seeds. Pull spaghetti strands free with a fork. Place squash in baking dish; ladle sauce over squash. Return to microwave and heat through. Sprinkle with cottage cheese. Serve with Applesauce Spice Muffins (page 219) and Strawberry-Banana Salad (page 72).

MAKES 4 SERVINGS
SERVING SIZE: 1 CUP SPAGHETTI SQUASH WITH 1 CUP OF SAUCE
CALORIES: 287 • CHOL.: 1 MG. • FAT: 12 G. • SODIUM: 324 MG.

Spaghetti with Bean Sauce

This entrée equals a meat dish because of the combination of beans and a grain (the wheat-based spaghetti).

Prepare Ahead

Pinto or Kidney beans*, Onion**

I medium ONION**, chopped

I CLOVE GARLIC, minced

2 Tbsp. VEGETABLE OIL

1-1/2 cups dried PINTO* or KIDNEY BEANS*, washed

I dried HOT PEPPER, crumbled

I tsp. SALT

1/2 tsp. PEPPER

4 cups WATER

1/4 tsp. crumbled DRIED BASIL

1/4 tsp. crumbled DRIED OREGANO

2 BEEF BOUILLON CUBES

I Tbsp. WHITE VINEGAR

I can (16 oz.) TOMATOES

I can (6 oz.) TOMATO PASTE

cooked SPAGHETTI

Sauté onion and garlic in oil for 5 minutes. Add beans, hot pepper, salt, pepper, and water. Cover and simmer until tender. Add remaining ingredients (except spaghetti) and simmer, uncovered, for about 1 hour, stirring occasionally. Serve sauce over cooked spaghetti, macaroni, or noodles.

TIP: Substitute canned beans for dry beans.

MAKES 10 SERVINGS

PASTA:

SERVING SIZE: 1/2 CUP

CALORIES: 100 • CHOL.: 0 • FAT: 0 • SODIUM: 1 MG.

SAUCE:

SERVING SIZE: 3/4 CUP

CALORIES: 165 • CHOL.: 0 • FAT: 3 G. • SODIUM: 1 MG.

---

*=Dangerous to some • **=Consume with caution • See pages 19-22 for more information

Spinach Pie

This recipe can also be served as an appetizer.

Specialty

Onion**

Crust (or use prepared crust):

> 3/4 cup ALL-PURPOSE FLOUR
> 1/8 tsp. SALT
> 3 Tbsp. REDUCED-CALORIE MARGARINE
> 2 Tbsp. ICE WATER

Preheat oven to 450 degrees. Combine flour and salt in medium-size bowl. Work in margarine with fork or pastry blender until mixture is crumbly. Add water and work until dough is formed. Pat dough into a disk. Place between 2 sheets waxed paper. Roll out into 11-inch circle. Fit into 7-1/2 inch fluted tart pan with removable bottom. Place square of aluminum foil in crust; add dried beans or rice to weight crust. Bake for 5 minutes. Remove foil and beans. Bake crust 10 minutes longer or until lightly browned. Remove from oven. Reduce oven temperature to 375 degrees.

Filling:

> NONSTICK COOKING SPRAY
> 1/4 cup chopped ONION**
> 1 CLOVE GARLIC, finely chopped
> 1 pkg. (10 oz.) frozen chopped SPINACH, thawed and drained well
> 1/2 cup LOW-FAT (1%) MILK
> 2 EGGS, beaten slightly
> 1/8 tsp SALT
> 1/4 tsp. PEPPER

Spray 10-inch nonstick skillet with cooking spray. Add onion and garlic, and sauté over medium heat for 2 minutes. Squeeze out excess liquid from spinach with paper toweling. Add spinach to skillet, then cook 1 minute; remove to medium-size bowl. Add milk, eggs, salt, and pepper to spinach mixture; stir to combine. Pour into crust.

continued...

*=Dangerous to some • **=Consume with caution • See pages 19-22 for more information

Bake at 375 degrees for 30 to 35 minutes or until center is set. Let stand about 10 minutes. Remove sides from pan. Cut pie into wedges to serve.

MAKES 4 SERVINGS

SERVING SIZE: 1/4 PIE

CALORIES: 200 • CHOL.: 145 MG. • FAT: 9 G. • SODIUM: 372 MG.

Spinach Potpourri

A very complete meal low in fat but high in flavor and nutrition.
The combination of onion, mushroom soup, potatoes, and spinach
can be ready in half an hour if planned ahead.

Quick and Easy

Mushrooms*, Onion**, Yogurt**

1/4 cup chopped RED ONION**
1 pkg. (10 oz.) frozen chopped SPINACH
2 Tbsp. WATER
1 can (10-3/4 oz.) condensed CREAM OF MUSHROOM SOUP*
1 soup can of WATER
1/8 tsp. GROUND NUTMEG
1/8 tsp. PEPPER
1/2 cup PLAIN NONFAT YOGURT**
1-1/2 cups peeled, diced, cooked POTATOES
1/2 cup SKIM MILK

In 2-quart covered saucepan over high heat, cook onion, spinach and
2 tablespoons water for 10 minutes or until vegetables are tender, stirring
occasionally. Reduce heat to medium. Blend in soup, soup can of water,
milk, nutmeg, and pepper. Cover; simmer 10 minutes. Stir in yogurt and
potatoes. Heat through. Do not boil.

TIP: To reduce sodium content, use low-sodium soup.

MAKES 6 SERVINGS
SERVING SIZE: 1 CUP
CALORIES: 142 • CHOL.: 2 MG. • FAT: 6 G. • SODIUM: 544 MG.

Vegetable Medley Quiche

Everyone seems to like quiche; this one sings with color,
as well as flavor and nutrition.

Specialty

1 small ZUCCHINI, sliced (about 1 cup)
1 small GREEN PEPPER, cut in strips (about 3/4 cup)
1 small RED PEPPER, cut in strips (about 3/4 cup)
1 tsp. MARGARINE
1 (9 inch) PASTRY CRUST
1 carton (8 oz.) EGG SUBSTITUTE, or 4 EGGS
1 cup SKIM MILK
1/4 tsp. BASIL LEAVES
1/8 tsp. PEPPER

Preheat oven to 375 degrees. In skillet over medium heat, cook zucchini, green pepper, and red pepper in margarine until crisp-tender, stirring occasionally. Spoon mixture into pastry crust. Mix egg substitute, skim milk, basil, and pepper; pour over vegetables. Bake for 50 to 55 minutes or until knife inserted in center comes out clean. Let stand 10 minutes before serving. Serve with a small side salad and a square of Honey Walnut Cake (page 246).

MAKES 8 SERVINGS
SERVING SIZE: 1/8 PIE WEDGE
CALORIES: 127 • CHOL.: 13 MG. • FAT: 8 G. • SODIUM: 211 MG

Vegetable Platter with Mustard Sauce

This dish focuses on two anti-cancer cruciferous ingredients.

Quick and Easy

1 small CAULIFLOWER, washed and trimmed but not cut up
1 pkg. (10 oz.) frozen BRUSSEL SPROUTS
1 Tbsp. FLOUR
1/2 cup SKIM MILK
1 Tbsp. DIJON MUSTARD
dash WHITE PEPPER
1/2 sweet RED PEPPER, cut into 2-inch julienne strips

In large saucepan over medium-high heat, steam whole cauliflower head in 1 inch of water 12 to 15 minutes or until tender. Remove to platter and keep warm. Cook Brussel sprouts according to package directions. In small saucepan over medium heat, combine flour, milk, mustard, and white pepper. Cook 5 minutes or until sauce thickens, stirring constantly. Arrange Brussel sprouts around cauliflower head on serving platter, with red pepper strips between Brussel sprouts. Pour sauce over cauliflower head.

Serve with Date-Nut Bread (page 209) and Caramel Custard (page 239).

MICROWAVE: On a microwave-safe serving platter, place cauliflower head upside down in center of platter. Arrange Brussel sprouts around cauliflower. Cover entire platter with plastic wrap. Microwave 3 minutes on high (100% power). Uncover platter, turn cauliflower right side up and re-cover with plastic wrap. Microwave 4-1/2 to 5 minutes more or until cauliflower and sprouts are tender. Let stand while preparing sauce. In 4-cup microwave-safe bowl, combine flour, milk, mustard, and white pepper. Microwave on high 1 to 1-1/2 minutes or until mixture thickens, stirring halfway through cooking. Uncover vegetables. Garnish with red pepper strips and top with mustard sauce.

MAKES 8 SERVINGS
SERVING SIZE: 3/4 CUP
CALORIES: 35 • CHOL.: 1 MG. • FAT: 1 G. • SODIUM: 50 MG.

*=Dangerous to some • **=Consume with caution • See pages 19-22 for more information

Meat
Entrées

Apple Stuffed Veal Rolls

Your grandmother prepared veal in a similar way with bread stuffing and called the dish "veal birds."

Specialty

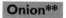

1/2 cup chopped ONION**
2 Tbsp. MARGARINE
3 cups day-old WHITE BREAD cubes
1 cup diced APPLE
dash PEPPER
1/2 cup WATER
1 lb. thinly sliced VEAL CUTLETS (4 large slices)
1 cup APPLE JUICE
1 Tbsp. CORNSTARCH
1/2 cup diagonally sliced CELERY, blanched
1/2 cup APPLE slices, blanched

Sauté onion in 1 tablespoon margarine until golden, about 5 minutes. Stir in bread cubes. Heat, stirring, until margarine is absorbed. Stir in diced apple, pepper, and 1/4 cup water.

Place 1/4 stuffing mixture (about 1/2 cup) near one edge of each cutlet. Roll up cutlets like a jelly roll. Melt remaining margarine in skillet over medium heat. Brown veal rolls on all sides. Add 1 cup apple juice to skillet. Cover and cook until veal is tender, about 15 to 20 minutes. Remove veal rolls to a warm platter.

Mix together remaining 1/4 cup water and cornstarch. Stir into pan juices. Cook until thickened, stirring constantly. Spoon over veal rolls and garnish platter with blanched celery and apple slices. Serve with Harlequin Slaw (page 66), whole wheat bread. and Cannoli Cream (page 238).

MAKES 4 SERVINGS
SERVING SIZE: 1 VEAL ROLL
CALORIES: 388 • CHOL.: 82 MG. • FAT: 16 G. • SODIUM: 312 MG.

Barbecued Pork on a Bun

*Now that pork is so much leaner, some nutritionists
refer to pork as "the other white meat."*

Quick and Easy • Prepare Ahead

Pork*, Onion**, Orange juice**, Oranges**

NON-STICK COOKING SPRAY
1 large ONION**, finely chopped
1 can (8 oz.) no-salt-added or regular TOMATO SAUCE
2 Tbsp. LIGHT BROWN SUGAR
1-2 Tbsp. WHITE VINEGAR
1 Tbsp. ORANGE JUICE**
2 tsp. PREPARED MUSTARD
1/8 tsp. PAPRIKA
1/8 tsp. GROUND HOT RED PEPPER
2 cups cooked SHREDDED PORK*
4 HAMBURGER BUNS, split and toasted
2 juice ORANGES**, cut into wedges

Spray medium size nonstick saucepan with cooking spray. Sauté onion in saucepan for 2 minutes or until tender. (Add a little water if necessary to prevent sticking.) Stir in tomato sauce, brown sugar, vinegar, orange juice, mustard, paprika, and red pepper. Bring to boiling. Lower heat; simmer, covered, 5 to 8 minutes or until thickened. Stir in pork.

To serve, spoon meat and sauce over toasted bun. Garnish with orange wedges and serve with Mandarin Salad (see Salads) and a Saucepan Butterscotch Brownie (see Desserts).

MAKES 4 SERVINGS
SERVING SIZE: 1/2 CUP PER BUN
CALORIES: 315 • CHOL.: 58 MG. • FAT: 5 G. • SODIUM: 292 MG.

*=Dangerous to some • **=Consume with caution • See pages 19-22 for more information

Beef Cube Steaks

Vegetables and cube steaks can be ready to eat in less time than it takes to eat them.

Quick and Easy

1 CLOVE GARLIC, minced
1/2 tsp. dried BASIL LEAVES
1/4 tsp. PEPPER
2 lean BEEF CUBED STEAKS (about 4 oz. each)
1 tsp. OLIVE OIL
2 small ZUCCHINI, thinly sliced, or 10 oz. frozen BROCCOLI
4 CHERRY TOMATOES, halved
1/4 tsp. SALT

Combine garlic, basil, and pepper; divide seasoning mixture in half. Press half of seasoning mixture evenly into both sides of beef cubed steaks; set aside.

Heat oil and remaining seasoning mixture in large nonstick frying pan over medium heat. Add zucchini or broccoli; cook and stir 2 to 3 minutes. Add tomatoes and cook 1 minute. Remove vegetables to warm platter and keep warm.

Increase heat to medium-high; add steaks. Cook steaks 3 to 4 minutes, turning once. Season steaks with salt. Serve with vegetables, relishes, Low-Salt Challa Bread (see Breads), Broccoli Pasta Salad (see Salads), and Baked Apple Crumble (see Desserts).

TIP: A butcher can mechanically tenderize most boneless cuts of meat, such as round steak.

MAKES 2 SERVINGS
SERVING SIZE: 1 STEAK AND 1/2 OF VEGETABLES
CALORIES: 279 • CHOL.: 77 MG. • FAT: 15 G. • SODIUM: 670 MG.

Beef Picadillo

*Add variety to your meal plans by preparing an
ethnic dish that is both tasty and healthy.*

Quick and Easy

Onion**

> 1-1/2 lbs. trimmed ROUND STEAK, cut into thin strips
> 1 Tbsp. MARGARINE
> 1 jar (12 oz.) SALSA, mild, medium, or hot
> 1 TOMATO, chopped
> 1/2 tsp. DRIED OREGANO LEAVES
> 2 Tbsp. instant, minced, or chopped ONION**
> 1/8 tsp. GARLIC POWDER

In large skillet over medium-high heat, cook steak strips in margarine about 5 minutes or until meat is no longer pink. Stir in salsa, tomato, oregano, onion, and garlic powder. Simmer for 10 minutes, stirring occasionally.

MICROWAVE: Melt margarine in microwave-safe dish. Mix steak strips with margarine. Cover dish. Cook on high (100% power) for 2 to 3 minutes or until meat is no longer pink. Stir after 1 to 1-1/2 minutes. Stir in salsa, tomato, oregano, onion, and garlic powder. Cook for 3 to 4 minutes on high, stirring occasionally.

Serve with Roasted Garlic Potatoes (see Side Dishes) and a tossed salad with Sprout Dressing (see Salads).

MAKES 6 SERVINGS
SERVING SIZE: 3/4 CUP
CALORIES: 202 • CHOL.: 70 MG. • FAT: 9 G. • SODIUM: 215 MG.

Cajun Jambalaya

Louisiana contributes this complete meal for a change from the ordinary casserole. Caution: You may want to start with less than 1/4 teaspoon of cayenne pepper! You can always add more, but wait a moment to see.

Specialty • Prepare Ahead

Onion**

1 Tbsp. VEGETABLE OIL
1/2 cup chopped ONIONS**
1/2 cup chopped GREEN PEPPER
1/2 cup chopped CELERY
1 can (16 oz.) WHOLE TOMATOES with juice
1 cup FAT-FREE CHICKEN BROTH
1/2 cup uncooked LONG GRAIN RICE
1/2 tsp. SALT
1/4 tsp. (or less) CAYENNE PEPPER
1 Tbsp. chopped PARSLEY
1/8 tsp. GROUND THYME
1-1/2 cups chopped, cooked CHICKEN (skin and fat removed)
1/2 cup chopped, cooked LEAN BEEF

Preheat a 2-quart saucepan over medium heat. Add oil, onions, peppers, and celery. Cook, stirring frequently, over medium heat until the onions are soft but not browned. Add tomatoes and juice, broth, rice, salt, pepper, parsley, and thyme to the vegetables. Cook uncovered 20 to 25 minutes, stirring frequently, until rice is cooked. If the mixture gets too dry, add hot water. Add chicken and beef and continue to cook until heated through. Serve hot.

MAKES 5 SERVINGS
SERVING SIZE: 1 CUP
CALORIES: 224 • CHOL.: 87 MG. • FAT: 23 G. • SODIUM: 551 MG.

---

*=Dangerous to some • **=Consume with caution • See pages 19-22 for more information

Chili Con Carne

Quick and Easy • Prepare Ahead

Beans*, Onion**

1/4 lb. LEAN GROUND BEEF
1/2 cup ONION**, chopped
1 CLOVE GARLIC, minced
generous dash GROUND CUMIN
1/2 cup canned TOMATOES AND GREEN CHILES
1 can (16. oz.) KIDNEY BEANS* in tomato sauce (no added salt)

Combine beef with onion, garlic, and cumin, and cook over medium heat in a medium saucepan until beef is browned. Stir to break up meat. Then add remaining ingredients; bring to a boil and reduce heat. Simmer, uncovered, for 10 minutes, stirring occasionally to blend flavors.

TIP: If Chili Con Carne is prepared ahead and stored in refrigerator overnight, the flavors blend and intensify.

MAKES 3 SERVINGS
SERVING SIZE: 1 CUP
CALORIES: 232 • CHOL.: 28 MG. • FAT: 5.2 G. • SODIUM: 72 MG.

---

*=Dangerous to some • **=Consume with caution • See pages 19-22 for more information

Beef Sandwich on Onion Bun

Preparing your own beef certainly lowers the percentage of fat you find in most fast foods.

Quick and Easy

Onion bun**

- 1 tsp. MUSTARD
- 1 ONION BUN**
- 2 oz. sliced LEAN BEEF
- 2 TOMATO slices
- 1 GREEN PEPPER, sliced thin

Spread mustard on bun. Pile beef and tomato on bun. Top with green pepper. Try this sandwich with Glazed Carrots (see page 170) and refreshing Smorgasbord Cheese Cake (see page 252).

MAKES 1 SERVING
SERVING SIZE: 1 SANDWICH
CALORIES: 374 • CHOL.: 35 MG. • FAT: 8 G. • SODIUM: 183 MG.

Citrus Chops

Because of changes in the pork industry, pork is no longer required to be cooked so long. Variation: substitute turkey ham for the pork.

Quick and Easy

Pork*, Onion**, Orange peel**, Orange juice**

I tsp. OIL
1/4 cup sliced GREEN ONION**
I Tbsp. grated ORANGE PEEL**
4 lean, trimmed PORK LOIN CHOPS*
1/2 cup ORANGE JUICE**
1/4 tsp. DRIED BASIL

Heat oil in large skillet. Add green onion and orange peel; sauté 3 to 4 minutes or until onion is almost tender. Remove onion and orange peel; set aside. Add pork chops and brown on both sides over medium heat; add onion and orange peel. Add orange juice and basil; cover and simmer for 10 minutes.

MICROWAVE: Omit oil; combine ingredients other than chops in a small bowl. Arrange chops in glass or ceramic dish with meaty parts to outside. Pour juice mixture over chops. Cover with plastic wrap; poke holes in plastic wrap. Microwave on medium (50% power) for 8 to 10 minutes. Turn dish or rearrange chops. Replace plastic wrap and microwave for another 8 to 10 minutes.

Complete the meal with Austrian Cooked Cabbage (see page 167) and Mock Rice Pudding (see page 248).

MAKES 4 SERVINGS
SERVING SIZE: I PORK CHOP
CALORIES: 222 • CHOL.: 73 MG. • FAT: 12 G. • SODIUM: 44 MG.

Favorite "Ham" Loaf

An old-time recipe, moist and tasty, that slices well.

Specialty • Prepare Ahead

"Ham" Loaf

I lb. ground SMOKED TURKEY HAM
1/2 lb. TURKEY SAUSAGE
1/2 lb. GROUND BEEF
1/2 tsp. SALT
1/4 chopped GREEN PEPPER
I EGG
2 Tbsp. MUSTARD
1/4 cup CATSUP
1/4 cup chopped PIMENTO
3/4 cup BREAD CRUMBS
3/4 cup MILK

Glaze

I cup drained, crushed PINEAPPLE
1/3 cup BROWN SUGAR

Preheat oven to 350 degrees. Combine "ham" ingredients and press into a large 8-1/2 x 4-1/2 loaf pan. Bake 1 hour or until loaf pulls away from edges. Mix pineapple with brown sugar. Ten minutes before the loaf is done, glaze with brown sugar topping. If desired; baste 2 or 3 times.

TIP: Slice cold "ham" loaf for delicious sandwiches.

MAKES 6 TO 8 SERVINGS
SERVING SIZE: I SLICE
CALORIES: 247 (APPROX.) • CHOL.: 92 MG. • FAT: 14 G. • SODIUM: 326 MG.

---

*=Dangerous to some • **=Consume with caution • See pages 19-22 for more information

Pork Stir-Fry

Quick and Easy

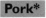
Pork*

1 Tbsp. VEGETABLE OIL

1 lb. trimmed, boneless PORK TENDERLOIN*,
cut crosswise into 1/4-inch strips

1 pkg. (16 oz.) frozen STIR-FRY VEGETABLES, thawed,
or 3 cups FRESH VEGETABLES cut into small pieces

SALT to taste

Heat oil over high heat in wok or large skillet. Quickly brown pork strips,
stirring constantly. Add vegetables; cover and steam for 3 to 5 minutes or
until vegetables are heated through but still crisp-tender. Fresh vegetables
will take longer to cook. Add salt; cook and stir one minute.

MAKES 4 SERVINGS

SERVING SIZE: 6 OUNCES

CALORIES: 186 • CHOL.: 74 MG. • FAT: 7 G. • SODIUM: 95 MG.

Flank Steak with Mushrooms

Broiling meat is one of the most successful ways to cut down on fat. Not only is the meat not cooked in fat, but the excess fat drips through the broiler rack.

Quick and Easy

Mushrooms*, Onion**

2 Tbsp. MARGARINE
1 lb. fresh MUSHROOMS*, sliced
1/4 cup chopped ONION**
1/3 cup APPLE JUICE
1 lb. FLANK STEAK
PARSLEY SPRIGS

Melt margarine in a large skillet over medium heat. Add mushrooms and onion; sauté, stirring occasionally, until tender and most of the mushroom liquid evaporates. Stir in apple juice and keep warm over low heat.

Broil steak 8 to 10 minutes on each side or to desired doneness. Cut into thin slices at an angle across grain. Serve topped with mushroom mixture and garnished with parsley sprigs.

MAKES 4 SERVINGS
SERVING SIZE: 4 OUNCES
CALORIES: 268 • CHOL.: 58 MG. • FAT: 16 G. • SODIUM: 99 MG.

Mexican Beef Stir-Fry

Fork-tender, full of flavor and nutritious; this colorful dish is served on a bed of lettuce.

Quick and Easy

Onion**

1 lb. well-trimmed TOP ROUND BEEF STEAK
1 Tbsp. VEGETABLE OIL
1 tsp. GROUND CUMIN
1 tsp. DRIED OREGANO LEAVES
1/8 tsp. GARLIC POWDER
1 RED BELL PEPPER, cut into thin strips
1 medium ONION**, cut into thin wedges
1 to 2 JALAPEÑO PEPPERS, cut into slivers
ROMAINE LETTUCE, cut 1/4-inch thick

Cut round steak into 1/8-inch thick strips. Combine oil, cumin, oregano, and garlic powder; reserve half. Heat half of the seasoned oil in large non-stick frying pan over medium-high heat until hot. Add red pepper, onion, and jalapeño pepper; stir-fry 2 to 3 minutes or until crisp-tender. Remove vegetables and set aside.

In same pan, stir-fry beef strips (half at a time) in reserved seasoned oil for 1 to 2 minutes. Return vegetables to pan and heat through. Serve beef mixture on a bed of lettuce.

MAKES 4 SERVINGS
SERVING SIZE: 4 OUNCES
CALORIES: 232 • CHOL.: 65 MG. • FAT: 12 G. • SODIUM: 34 MG.

Pork Tenderloin with Orange Marmalade Sauce

The popular kiwifruit is even more laden with vitamin C than oranges.

Quick and Easy

Pork*, Orange**, Orange marmalade**

1 lb. PORK TENDERLOIN*, trimmed and cut into 8 pieces
CAYENNE PEPPER, to taste
1 Tbsp. MARGARINE
6 Tbsp. ORANGE MARMALADE**
2 Tbsp. WHITE VINEGAR
1 Tbsp. KETCHUP
1/2 tsp. HORSERADISH
1/8 tsp. GARLIC POWDER
2 KIWIFRUIT, peeled, thinly sliced
ORANGE* segments (optional)

Press each pork tenderloin slice to 1-inch thickness. Lightly sprinkle both sides of each slice with cayenne pepper. Heat margarine in large heavy skillet over medium-high heat. Add pork slices; cook 5 to 7 minutes on each side, or until meat is no longer pink inside.

Combine orange marmalade, vinegar, ketchup, horseradish, and garlic powder in small saucepan. Simmer over low heat about 5 minutes, stirring occasionally. Place cooked pork slices on warm serving plate. Spoon sauce over pork; top each slice with a kiwi slice. Garnish with remaining kiwi slices and orange segments, if desired.

MICROWAVE: Prepare pork slices as above. Melt margarine in large microwave-safe dish; add pork slices. Cover and cook 6 to 8 minutes on high (100% power). Turn dish and meat every 3 minutes. Combine marmalade, vinegar, ketchup, horseradish, and garlic powder in small bowl. Microwave 1 to 2 minutes, stirring occasionally. Place pork slices on warm serving platter and garnish and serve as above.

MAKES 4 SERVINGS
SERVING SIZE: 4 OUNCES
CALORIES: 267 • CHOL.: 74 MG. • FAT: 7 G. • SODIUM: 136 MG.

*=Dangerous to some • **=Consume with caution • See pages 19-22 for more information

Savory Beef Burgers

Mama mia! What a burger! And, of course,
have at hand the ketchup, etc., for burger purists.

Quick and Easy

Onion**

1 lb. EXTRA LEAN GROUND BEEF
2 Tbsp. INSTANT MINCED ONION**
1 Tbsp. DIJON MUSTARD
3/4 tsp. DRIED ITALIAN SEASONING
1/4 tsp. GROUND CUMIN
1/4 tsp. CRACKED BLACK PEPPER
1/2 tsp. salt
4 TOMATO slices, 1/4-inch thick
4-8 LETTUCE LEAVES
4 thin RED ONION RINGS**
4 BURGER BUNS

Combine ground beef, onion, mustard, Italian seasoning, cumin, pepper, and salt. Mix lightly but thoroughly. Divide beef mixture into 4 equal portions and form into patties. Place patties on rack in broiler pan so surface of meat is 3 to 4 inches from heat. Broil 8 to 10 minutes, turning once. Assemble burger submarine sandwich style with tomato, lettuce, and onion. Serve immediately.

MICROWAVE: Prepare ground beef mixture as above. Place patties in a microwave-safe baking dish. Cook on high (100% power) 8 minutes, turning dish after first 4 minutes. Assemble and serve as above.

MAKES 4 SERVINGS
SERVING SIZE: 1 BURGER
CALORIES: 239 • CHOL.: 81 MG. • FAT: 13 G. • SODIUM: 90 MG.

Savory Brushed Steak

Flank steak is another lean steak; flank steak may be a tough or tender steak depending on how the animal was exercised, age, type, etc. Note the market's tenderness category.

Onion**, Lemon juice**

1/4 cup MARGARINE
1/4 cup minced ONION**
1/4 cup LEMON JUICE**
1/2 tsp. OREGANO LEAVES
1/4 tsp. MARJORAM LEAVES
1/4 tsp. THYME LEAVES
1/4 tsp. PEPPER
1 small CLOVE GARLIC, minced
2 lbs. FLANK STEAK, 1-1/2 to 2 inches thick

Melt margarine and mix in onion, lemon juice, oregano, marjoram, thyme, pepper, and garlic. Transfer sauce to a heavy plastic bag. Place steak in bag and seal closed. Turn bag to coat meat evenly with marinade. Let stand at room temperature 30 minutes.

Remove meat from bag; place meat on broiling rack. Remove excess marinade from bag. Brush surface of meat with half the marinade. Broil for 7 minutes; turn and brush with remaining marinade. Broil about 7 to 8 minutes longer or to desired doneness.

MAKES 8 SERVINGS
SERVING SIZE: 4 OUNCES
CALORIES: 256 • CHOL.: 58 MG. • FAT: 18 G. • SODIUM: 118 MG.

Spicy Pot Roast with Dumplings

A dish to prepare when you have the energy and the time.

Specialty

Curry powder*, Onion**

Pot Roast:

2 Tbsp. MARGARINE

3 lbs. POT ROAST OF BEEF

1 can (16 oz.) LOW-SODIUM TOMATOES, undrained

2 cups sliced ONIONS**

2 tsp. CURRY POWDER*

1 tsp. SUGAR

Dumplings:

1-1/2 cups ALL-PURPOSE FLOUR

1 Tbsp. LOW-SODIUM BAKING POWDER

1 Tbsp. MARGARINE

1 cup SKIM MILK

2 Tbsp. finely chopped ONION**

2 Tbsp. chopped PARSLEY

2 Tbsp. PIMENTO pieces

1 cup HOT WATER

In a large, heavy pan, melt margarine over medium-high heat. Add beef and brown on all sides. Add tomatoes and sliced onions; bring to a boil. Reduce heat, cover and simmer for 2 hours. Stir in curry powder and sugar. Cover and cook an additional 1/2 hour. Place roast on serving platter and keep warm.

DUMPLINGS: Combine flour and baking powder in a small bowl. Cut in margarine using a pastry blender or 2 knives. Stir in milk, chopped onion, parsley, and pimento pieces until moistened.

Add hot water to gravy mixture in pot; bring to a boil. Drop batter by tablespoonfuls into boiling gravy in pot. Cover, and cook over low heat
continued...

---

for 15 minutes. Arrange dumplings around pot roast on platter. Slice roast and serve with tomato gravy.

MAKES 12 SERVINGS
SERVING SIZE: 1 CUP
CALORIES: 267 • CHOL.: 69 MG. • FAT 9 G. • SODIUM: 117 MG.

Tacos

A Mexican specialty so popular and tasty that it's had a restaurant chain named for it. To reduce calorie count, use soft taco shells that haven't been fried.

Quick and Easy

Onion**

1 lb. EXTRA-LEAN GROUND BEEF
1 medium ONION**, chopped
2 CLOVES GARLIC, minced
2 tsp. CHILI POWDER
2 tsp. DRIED OREGANO
1/4 tsp. SALT
6 drops HOT PEPPER SAUCE
1/2 tsp. GROUND CUMIN
1/2 cup TOMATO SAUCE
6 TACO SHELLS
1 cup shredded LETTUCE
1/2 cup chopped TOMATOES
6 Tbsp. LOW-FAT COTTAGE CHEESE

Cook crumbled ground beef in a large skillet over medium heat until it begins to lose its pink color. Add onion and garlic. Cook until onion is translucent. Drain fat off. Add chili powder, oregano, salt, hot pepper sauce, cumin, and tomato sauce, and simmer about 10 minutes.

Fill each taco shell with 1/3 cup of cooked mixture. Top with shredded lettuce, chopped tomato, and 1 tablespoon cottage cheese.

MAKES 6 SERVINGS
SERVING SIZE: 1 TACO
CALORIES: 230 • CHOL.: 60 MG. • FAT: 9 G. • SODIUM: 210 MG.

Texas Meatloaf

Here's a recipe the whole family will enjoy. You can bake it in four small individual loaves or double the recipe to have an extra loaf for the freezer.

Specialty • Prepare Ahead

Onion**

NON-STICK OIL COOKING SPRAY

2 Tbsp. CORN OIL

1 GREEN PEPPER, coarsely chopped

1 large ONION**, chopped

3 CLOVES GARLIC, minced or pressed

1 1/2 lbs. LEAN GROUND BEEF

2 EGG WHITES, or 2 EGGS, or 1/4 cup EGG SUBSTITUTE

3/4 cup OLD-FASHIONED OATS

3/4 cup BARBECUE SAUCE, divided

1 can (4 oz.) chopped GREEN CHILES, undrained

Preheat oven to 350 degrees. Spray 8-1/2 x 4-1/2 x 2-1/2 inch loaf pan with cooking spray. In large skillet heat corn oil over medium heat. Add pepper, onion, and garlic. Sauté 4 to 5 minutes or until tender. Remove from heat. In large bowl combine ground beef, egg whites, oats, 1/2 cup barbecue sauce and chiles. Stir in cooked vegetables. Spoon into loaf pan. Bake 1 hour. Drain off excess liquid. Invert loaf onto serving platter. Spoon remaining 1/4 cup barbecue sauce over loaf. Let stand 10 minutes before slicing. Serve with Lemon-Herb Twice-Baked Potato (see page 175).

MAKES 8 SERVINGS

SERVING SIZE: 4 OUNCES

CALORIES: 260 • CHOL.: 55 MG. • FAT: 12 G. • SODIUM: 410 MG.

Veal Scallopini

If veal is difficult to find in your market, substitute beef cube steak. The beef flavor is a little more "hearty" than beef, but both veal and cube steak are lower in fat content than most beef cuts.

Quick and Easy

Mushrooms*

3 Tbsp. MARGARINE
1/2 lb. fresh MUSHROOMS*, sliced
1/4 cup ALL-PURPOSE FLOUR
1/8 tsp. PEPPER
1 lb. thinly sliced VEAL CUTLETS
1/4 cup WHITE VINEGAR
1 Tbsp. WATER
chopped PARSLEY

Melt 1 tablespoon margarine in a large skillet over medium heat. Add mushrooms and sauté until tender; remove from pan.

Combine flour and pepper; coat veal with flour mixture. Melt remaining margarine in nonstick skillet and brown veal, a few pieces at a time, until done; remove from pan. Add vinegar and water to skillet, stirring until liquid is slightly thickened. Return veal and mushrooms to pan to heat through. Arrange on a serving platter and garnish with chopped parsley.

MAKES 4 SERVINGS
SERVING SIZE: 4 OUNCES
CALORIES: 302 • CHOL.: 81 MG. • FAT: 18 G. • SODIUM: 153 MG.

Poultry Entrées

Barbecued Chicken

A chicken dish that tastes good hot or cold. May also be frozen and reheated later.

Prepare Ahead

Onion**

2 Tbsp. MARGARINE

1/4 cup chopped ONION**

2 Tbsp. diced GREEN PEPPER

1/2 cup LOW-SODIUM TOMATO JUICE

1/2 cup (4 cubes) frozen LOW-SODIUM TOMATO BASE
(see Sauces, Toppings) or BARBECUE SAUCE

2 Tbsp. firmly packed DARK BROWN SUGAR

2 Tbsp. WHITE VINEGAR

1/4 tsp. DRY MUSTARD

1/8 tsp. GARLIC POWDER

1/8 tsp. PEPPER

1 3-lb. CHICKEN, cut up

In small saucepan, melt margarine over medium heat. Add onion and green pepper; sauté until tender. Stir in tomato juice, tomato base, brown sugar, vinegar, dry mustard, garlic powder, and pepper. Reduce heat to low and simmer, stirring occasionally, until very thick, about 30 minutes. Place in blender or food processor; process until very smooth.

Remove all visible fat and loose skin from chicken pieces. Arrange chicken on broiler pan and brush with prepared sauce. Broil 5 to 6 inches from heat source for 20 to 25 minutes. Turn pieces, brush again with remaining sauce, and broil for 20 to 25 minutes more or until done. Serve hot or cold. Add Apple-Glazed Acorn Squash (see page 166) and Whole Grain Muffins (see page 221) to round out this meal.

MAKES 8 SERVINGS

SERVING SIZE: 1/3 - 1/2 POUND PER PERSON

CALORIES: 180 • CHOL.: 66 MG. • FAT: 4 G. • SODIUM: 105 MG.

Broiled Chicken Mexicana

Plain, white chicken breasts can become boring; here is another way to prepare white-meat poultry.

Quick and Easy • Prepare Ahead

Lime juice**, Green onions**

2 whole boneless, skinless CHICKEN BREASTS (about 1 lb.)
1/4 cup LIME JUICE**
1/4 cup VEGETABLE OIL
1/4 cup chopped CILANTRO or PARSLEY
2 CLOVES GARLIC, minced or pressed
2 Tbsp. chopped, pickled JALAPEÑO PEPPERS
1/4 tsp. SALT
2 cups chopped TOMATOES
1/2 cup sliced GREEN ONIONS**

Place chicken breasts in shallow baking dish. In small bowl combine lime juice, vegetable oil, cilantro, garlic, peppers, and salt. Pour half over chicken. Cover and marinate at room temperature 30 minutes.

Meanwhile, prepare salsa by adding tomatoes and green onions to mixture remaining in bowl. Set aside. Remove chicken from marinade, reserving 2 tablespoons for basting. Discard remaining marinade. Broil or grill chicken 6 inches from heat, basting occasionally, 15 to 20 minutes or until done. Serve with salsa. Delicious with Mexican Corn (see page 176) and Cashew Raisin Nuggets (see page 241).

MAKES 4 SERVINGS
SERVING SIZE: 1/3 - 1/2 POUND PER PERSON
CALORIES: 220 • CHOL.: 65 MG. • FAT: 10 G. • SODIUM: 330 MG.

---

*=Dangerous to some • **=Consume with caution • See pages 19-22 for more information

Chicken à la Divan

Tasting very French, delicate but rich in flavor, this dish is still low in calories, cholesterol, and fat.

Easy • Prepare Ahead

---

3 cups cooked fresh BROCCOLI SPEARS,
   or 2 (10 oz.) pkgs. frozen BROCCOLI SPEARS, cooked and drained

1-1/2 lbs. sliced cooked CHICKEN BREAST

3 Tbsp. MARGARINE

3 Tbsp. ALL-PURPOSE FLOUR

1-1/2 cups SKIM MILK

1/2 cup EGG SUBSTITUTE or 2 EGGS

2 Tbsp. WHITE VINEGAR

PAPRIKA

Preheat oven to 350 degrees. Arrange broccoli in the bottom of a shallow 2-quart baking dish or 6 individual baking dishes. Place chicken slices over broccoli. Cover with foil and bake for 20 minutes or until hot. Melt margarine in saucepan. Blend in flour; cook over low heat, stirring, until smooth and bubbly. Remove from heat and gradually stir in milk. Return to heat and bring to boil, stirring constantly. Gradually blend about half the hot mixture into egg substitute, then combine with remaining hot mixture. Stir in vinegar. Spoon sauce over chicken and broccoli; sprinkle lightly with paprika and serve.

MICROWAVE: In 2-quart microwave-proof shallow baking dish, arrange broccoli. Place chicken slices over broccoli; cover. Microwave on high (100% power) for 5 to 7 minutes or until hot, rotating dish 1/4 turn after 3 minutes. Let stand, covered, while preparing sauce. In 1-quart microwave-proof glass measure, microwave margarine and flour on high for 2 minutes, stirring after 1 minute. Gradually stir in milk. Microwave on high for 3-1/2 to 4-1/2 minutes, stirring every minute until thick and bubbly. Blend into egg substitute and proceed as above.

MAKES 6 SERVINGS
SERVING SIZE: 1 CUP
CALORIES: 192 • CHOL.: 49 MG. • FAT: 6 G. • SODIUM: 130 MG.

*=Dangerous to some • **=Consume with caution • See pages 19-22 for more information

Chicken and Mushroom Dijon

This recipe will please your taste buds; yet is so quick and easy to prepare.

Quick and Easy

2 Tbsp. MARGARINE
2 whole boneless skinless CHICKEN BREASTS, cut in half (about 1 lb.)
2 cups sliced fresh MUSHROOMS*
1 small ONION**, chopped
2/3 cup CHICKEN BROTH
1 tsp. CORNSTARCH
1 Tbsp. DIJON MUSTARD

In large skillet melt margarine over medium heat. Add chicken; sauté, turning frequently, 5 to 7 minutes or until done. Remove chicken. Add mushrooms and onion to skillet; sauté 3 minutes.

In small bowl, stir chicken broth and cornstarch until smooth; whisk in mustard. Stir into mushroom mixture. Stirring constantly, bring to boil and boil 1 minute. Serve over chicken.

Add Grilled Zucchini (see Side Dishes) and Strawberry-Banana Salad (see Salads) to complete your meal.

MAKES 4 SERVINGS
SERVING SIZE: 1/2 CHICKEN BREAST
CALORIES: 210 • CHOL.: 65 MG. • FAT: 8 G. • SODIUM: 410 MG.

Chicken Breasts with Mushroom-Apple Juice Sauce

A complete, tasty meal with a different flavor.
The mushrooms add texture and the parsley color contrast.

Easy • Prepare Ahead

Mushrooms*, Onion**

2 Tbsp. ALL-PURPOSE FLOUR

1/8 tsp. PEPPER

2 CHICKEN BREASTS, skinned, boned and split in half (about 1 lb. boneless)

2 Tbsp. MARGARINE

2 cups thinly sliced MUSHROOMS*

1/4 cup chopped ONION**

1 cup APPLE JUICE

1/4 cup minced PARSLEY

2 cups hot COOKED RICE (prepared without added salt)

Combine flour and pepper; coat chicken breasts with mixture. Shake off and reserve excess flour.

Heat margarine in a large skillet over medium heat. Brown chicken on both sides, then remove from skillet. Add mushrooms and onion to skillet. Sauté until tender and golden. Stir in reserved flour; blend in apple juice. Bring to a boil, stirring frequently. Return chicken to skillet with 2 tablespoons parsley. Cover; reduce heat and simmer for 25 minutes or until chicken is tender.

Serve over rice; garnish with remaining parsley.

MAKES 4 SERVINGS

SERVING SIZE: 1/2 CHICKEN BREAST AND 1/2 CUP RICE

CALORIES: 316 • CHOL.: 66 MG. • FAT: 7 G. • SODIUM: 127 MG.

Chicken Cacciatore

The wonderful aroma of the onion, spices, and chicken throughout the house will have everyone ready for this great Italian dish.

Specialty • Prepare Ahead

Onion**

3 whole CHICKEN BREASTS, split and skinned (about 3 lbs.)

3 Tbsp. MARGARINE

1 cup sliced ONION**

1/2 cup diced GREEN PEPPER

1 CLOVE GARLIC, crushed

1/2 tsp. OREGANO LEAVES

1/2 tsp. BASIL LEAVES

1/4 tsp. PEPPER

1/4 tsp. CELERY SEED

1 BAY LEAF

1 (16 oz.) can LOW-SODIUM TOMATOES, undrained

2 Tbsp. ALL-PURPOSE FLOUR

chopped PARSLEY

Remove fat from chicken. Melt margarine in skillet; brown both sides of chicken. Remove from skillet. Add onion, green pepper, and garlic to skillet. Sauté until onion is tender. Stir in seasonings and tomatoes. Add chicken; bring to boil. Cover; reduce heat and simmer for 1 hour, turning chicken halfway through cooking. Remove bay leaf. Remove chicken to serving platter.

Blend together flour and small amount of sauce from skillet; stir into mixture in skillet. Cook until thickened, about 3 minutes. Pour over chicken; garnish with parsley.

Add a crusty bread and a tossed salad. Top off the meal with Cannoli Cream (see page 238).

MAKES 6 SERVINGS

SERVING SIZE: 1 CUP

CALORIES: 213 • CHOL.: 66 MG. • FAT: 7 G. • SODIUM: 132 MG.

*=Dangerous to some • **=Consume with caution • See pages 19-22 for more information

Chicken Egg Sandwich

This recipe makes a hearty, juicy sandwich.

Quick and Easy

1/2 cup hard-cooked EGG SUBSTITUTE, hard cooked,
 or 2 EGGS, hard-cooked and sliced
8 slices salt-free WHOLE WHEAT BREAD
3 Tbsp. MARGARINE
4 LETTUCE LEAVES
3/4 lb. sliced cooked CHICKEN BREAST
1 medium TOMATO, sliced
PEPPER
4 slices WHOLE WHEAT BREAD

To hard cook egg substitute, pour into a heavy 8-inch skillet. Cover tightly. Cook over very low heat 10 minutes. Remove from heat. Allow to stand, covered, for 10 minutes.

Spread one side of bread slices with margarine. Layer lettuce leaves, eggs or egg substitute, chicken and tomato slices on 2 slices of bread. Sprinkle lightly with pepper. Top with remaining bread. Cut into quarters and serve.

MAKES 4 SERVINGS
SERVING SIZE: 1 SANDWICH
CALORIES: 397 • CHOL.: 24 MG. • FAT: 14 G. • SODIUM: 138 MG.

Chicken in Minced Parsley Sauce

Here's a delicious twist on those chicken breasts you've been eating.
The multicolored peppers are also a treat to the eye.

Prepare Ahead

Onion**

1 Tbsp. OLIVE OIL
1 each small GREEN, RED and YELLOW PEPPERS, sliced into 1/4-inch rings
6 boneless, skinless CHICKEN BREASTS (1-1/2 lbs. total)
2 cups (two 8-oz. cans) TOMATO SAUCE
1/2 cup minced fresh PARSLEY
1/2 cup coarsely chopped ONION**
1 medium GARLIC CLOVE, crushed
1/8 tsp. SALT

In 12-inch skillet, sauté pepper rings in oil until slightly tender. Remove; drain on paper towels. Brown chicken breasts in remaining oil in skillet. Keep warm.

In blender, process tomato sauce, parsley, onion, garlic, and salt until smooth. Pour over chicken in skillet. Heat to boiling; reduce heat; boil gently 5 minutes or until chicken is tender. Place chicken breasts on serving platter; arrange peppers on top. Serve with remaining sauce.

MAKES 6 SERVINGS
SERVING SIZE: 1 CHICKEN BREAST
CALORIES: 180 • CHOL.: 66 MG. • FAT: 4 G. • SODIUM: 459 MG.

Chicken Pot Pie

Specialty • Prepare Ahead

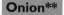

Onion**

1 BROILER-FRYER CHICKEN, cut up (3-1/2 lbs.)
1/2 cup sliced ONION**
1/2 cup chopped CELERY
1/8 tsp. PEPPER
dash POULTRY SEASONING
1 cup WATER
1/2 cup chopped WHITE ONION**
1 medium POTATO, peeled and cubed
2 medium CARROTS, cut in chunks
1/4 cup ALL-PURPOSE FLOUR
1/4 cup SKIM MILK
1 (10 oz.) pkg. frozen CUT GREEN BEANS
1/4 cup chopped PARSLEY
SINGLE CRUST FLAKY PASTRY (see Desserts, Sweets)

Remove visible fat from chicken. In a large heavy pan, combine chicken, sliced onion, celery, pepper, poultry seasoning, and water. Bring to a boil; reduce heat. Cover and simmer for 30 minutes or until chicken is tender. Remove chicken from broth; discard skin and bones, cutting meat into 1/2-inch cubes. Chill chicken and broth, separately. Discard fat from chilled broth and bring to a boil over medium-high heat; add chopped onions, potato, and carrots. Reduce heat and cook until vegetables are tender-crisp. Blend flour with skim milk. Add a little broth to the flour mixture; mix well. Quickly stir flour mixture into broth and vegetables. Bring to a boil over high heat, stirring constantly. Reduce heat to medium low; add green beans, parsley, and cubed chicken. Simmer for 2 minutes. Preheat oven to 425 degrees. Pour chicken mixture into a 2-quart shallow baking dish. Prepare pastry. Roll out to fit top of dish and prick with fork. Arrange pastry over chicken mixture; flute edges, pressing crust firmly to edge of baking dish. Bake for 20 to 25 minutes or until crust is golden brown.

MAKES 8 SERVINGS
SERVING SIZE: 1/8 OF POT PIE
CALORIES: 329 • CHOL.: 63 MG. • FAT: 13 G. • SODIUM: 145 MG.

*=Dangerous to some • **=Consume with caution • See pages 19-22 for more information

Chicken Scampi

*"Wok" your way to health with this tasty, complete meal
for dinner (but it also makes a great second-day lunch)!*

Prepare Ahead

Onion**, Lemon juice**

4 tsp. OLIVE OIL

1 large ONION**, sliced

1 large GREEN PEPPER, seeded and cut into bite-sized pieces

2 whole CHICKEN BREASTS, boned, skinned and cut into bite-sized pieces

16 oz. frozen BROCCOLI, chopped into bite-sized pieces

juice from 1/2 LEMON**, or 1 Tbsp. bottled LEMON JUICE**

1/2 tsp. SALT

1/2 tsp. PEPPER

8 oz. LINGUINE

PAPRIKA

Heat olive oil in large frying pan or wok over medium-high heat. Add onion, green pepper, and chicken; stir-fry about 5 minutes, or until meat changes color. Add broccoli and stir-fry for about 4 minutes, or until tender. Sprinkle with lemon juice, salt, and pepper.

Cook linguine in large pot of boiling water for 9 minutes or until tender; drain. Place linguine in large serving dish. Top with chicken-vegetable mixture; sprinkle with paprika.

MAKES 4 SERVINGS

SERVING SIZE: 1-1/2 CUPS

CALORIES: 485 • CHOL.: 70 MG. • FAT: 10 G. • SODIUM: 30 MG.

Herb Roasted Turkey & Potatoes
A hearty meat and potatoes dish.

Easy • Specialty

Onion salt**

1-1/2 lbs. fresh boneless TURKEY BREAST ROAST, skinned
1/8 tsp. GARLIC POWDER
4 RED or WHITE POTATOES
1/4 tsp. ONION SALT**
3/4 tsp. DRIED OREGANO LEAVES
2 Tbsp. MARGARINE, melted
PAPRIKA

Preheat oven to 350 degrees. Sprinkle garlic powder over surface of turkey. Place turkey in 9 x 9-inch pan; quarter potatoes and place around roast. Combine onion salt and oregano; sprinkle roast with 2/3 of the onion-oregano mixture. Drizzle margarine over potatoes and sprinkle with remaining onion-oregano mixture and paprika. Bake 1-1/2 hours or until internal temperature reaches 170 degrees.

MICROWAVE: Prepare roast and potatoes as above. Place in microwave-proof baking dish. Microwave on medium (50% power) for 18 to 20 minutes or until the internal temperature reaches 170 degrees. Turn dish every 5 to 6 minutes.

Complement this meal with Festive Cranberry Sauce (see page 203) and Glazed Carrots (see page 170).

MAKES 6 SERVINGS
SERVING SIZE: 6 OUNCES
CALORIES: 280 • CHOL.: 68 MG. • FAT: 12 G. • SODIUM: 69 MG.

Lemon Chicken

Lemon and chicken seem to have an affinity for each other.

Easy • Prepare Ahead

Lemon juice**

1/2 cup LEMON JUICE**
1/8 tsp. GARLIC POWDER
1/2 tsp. DRIED ROSEMARY
1/2 tsp. DRIED PARSLEY
1 BROILER OR FRYER CHICKEN, cut in parts and skinned

Combine lemon juice, garlic powder, rosemary, and parsley in a medium-sized glass or plastic dish. Roll chicken parts in lemon mixture to coat. Cover and refrigerate chicken in marinade 10 to 20 minutes. Drain chicken, reserving lemon mixture. Broil or grill chicken 5 to 6 inches from heat, brushing with reserved lemon mixture. Continue cooking and basting until chicken is fork tender, about 35 to 45 minutes.

MICROWAVE: Prepare lemon mixture and chicken as above. After marinating chicken, place in microwave-safe dish, and cover with vented plastic wrap; microwave on medium (50% power) for 16 to 20 minutes. Turn or rearrange chicken pieces so that less cooked parts are to the outside. Baste with reserved lemon mixture; replace wrap and continue cooking until chicken is fork tender, about 7 to 10 minutes more.

Peas seem to be a natural to serve with lemon chicken or try Green Beans Delicious (see page 171).

MAKES 4 SERVINGS
SERVING SIZE: 1/4 CHICKEN
CALORIES: 228 • CHOL.: 102 MG. • FAT: 8 G. • SODIUM: 77 MG.

*=Dangerous to some • **=Consume with caution • See pages 19-22 for more information

Microwave Chicken Italiano

Another one-dish, low-calorie meal with zucchini,
carrots, and onion. Good as a leftover, too.

Prepare Ahead

Onion**

8 CHICKEN BREAST HALVES, boned and skinned (2-1/2 to 3 lbs.)
1-1/2 tsp. SEASONED SALT, divided
1/8 tsp. PEPPER
1 medium ONION**, sliced
1 cup (2 medium) thinly sliced CARROTS
2/3 cup (6-oz. can) TOMATO PASTE
1 can (10-1/2 oz.) CHICKEN BROTH
1/4 cup WATER
1/2 tsp. DRIED OREGANO LEAVES, crushed
1/2 tsp. DRIED BASIL
1 large GARLIC CLOVE, minced
pinch crushed RED PEPPER FLAKES (optional)
1 cup (1 medium) julienned ZUCCHINI

In 13 x 9 x 2-inch microwave-safe dish, place chicken breasts; season with 1 teaspoon seasoned salt and pepper. Distribute onion and carrot over chicken pieces; set aside.

In small bowl, blend tomato paste, chicken broth, water, remaining 1/2 teaspoon seasoned salt, oregano, basil, garlic, and red pepper flakes, if desired. Pour over chicken, onion, and carrots; cover, venting edge. Microwave on high (100% power) for 10 minutes. Turn chicken pieces over and rearrange in dish. Cover and cook additional 7 minutes. Mix in zucchini; cover and cook 5 minutes or until chicken is cooked. Let stand, covered, 5 minutes before serving.

MAKES 8 SERVINGS
SERVING SIZE: 1 CUP
CALORIES: 244 • CHOL.: 107 MG. • FAT: 3 G. • SODIUM: 777 MG.

Orange Chicken Crepes

A festive dish for any meal—the seedless green grapes
make a special effect and taste contrast.

Specialty • Prepare Ahead

2 Tbsp. chopped CELERY
2 Tbsp. chopped ONION**
1 Tbsp. MARGARINE
1/4 cup ALL-PURPOSE FLOUR
dash PEPPER
1-2/3 cups SKIM MILK
2 Tbsp. minced PARSLEY
1/4 cup ORANGE JUICE**
1-1/2 cups chopped cooked CHICKEN
3/4 cup SEEDLESS GREEN GRAPES, halved
8 PREPARED CREPES (see below)

Preheat oven to 350 degrees. Saute celery and onion in margarine 2 to 3 minutes. Stir in flour and pepper. Gradually stir in milk. Bring to a boil, stirring constantly; cook 1 minute more. Remove from heat; stir in parsley and orange juice.

Mix half the prepared sauce with chicken and grapes. Spoon chicken mixture on crepes; roll up and place in a greased 11 x 7 x 1-1/2 inch baking dish. Pour remaining sauce over crepes. Bake for 20 minutes or until hot. Garnish with additional grapes, if desired.

Crepes

Mix 2/3 cup skim milk, 2/3 cup all-purpose flour and 6 tablespoons egg substitute until smooth. Mix in 1 tablespoon melted margarine. Chill batter 30 minutes.

Melt 1/2 tablespoon margarine and lightly brush a heated 8-inch skillet. Pour in 2 tablespoons prepared batter; tip pan to spread mixture evenly. Cook until bottom is sightly browned. Turn and brown other side. Turn out onto waxed paper. Repeat, brushing skillet with melted margarine as needed.

continued...

*=Dangerous to some • **=Consume with caution • See pages 19-22 for more information

MICROWAVE: In 1-quart microwave-proof glass measure, place celery, onion, margarine, flour, and pepper. Microwave on high (100% power) for 1 minute. Gradually stir in milk. Microwave on high for 6 to 8 minutes, stirring every 2 minutes until thick and bubbly. Stir in parsley and orange juice. Prepare chicken mixture and fill crepes. Place crepes in greased 11 x 7 x 1-1/2 inch microwave-proof baking dish. Pour remaining sauce over crepes. Cover, and microwave on high for 8 to 10 minutes, rotating a half turn after 4 minutes. Let stand 5 minutes before serving.

MAKES 4 SERVINGS
SERVING SIZE: 2 CREPES
CALORIES: 368 • CHOL.: 50 MG. • FAT: 11 G. • SODIUM: 211 MG.

Grilled Piquante Chicken

For a taste bud treat try grilled poultry. Serve with julienne potatoes, zucchini, and red pepper strips in foil packets.

Easy • Prepare Ahead

1 cup THICK SALSA
2 packs SUGAR SUBSTITUTE
4 tsp. DIJON MUSTARD
4 CHICKEN BREASTS, skinned, boned, and cut in half

Mix salsa, sugar substitute, and mustard. Marinate chicken breasts in this mixture for 2 hours in refrigerator.

When coals have turned white, place chicken breasts on barbecue grill. Using a long-handled brush and wearing mitts, brush on marinade while grilling. Turn after about 5 minutes. They should be done in 10 to 15 minutes.

MAKES 8 SERVINGS
SERVING SIZE: 1/2 CHICKEN BREAST
CALORIES: 154 • CHOL.: 73 MG. • FAT: 3 G. • SODIUM: 217 MG.

*=Dangerous to some • **=Consume with caution • See pages 19-22 for more information

Oven-Crisp Chicken Breasts

This recipe duplicates the flavor and crunch of
deep-fat fried chicken without all the fat and calories.

Prepare Ahead

---

    8 boneless CHICKEN BREASTS (about 2 lbs.)
    2 EGG WHITES
    1/2 cup SKIM MILK
    1/2 cup ALL-PURPOSE FLOUR
    1 Tbsp. PAPRIKA
    1 tsp. DRIED BASIL LEAVES
    1/2 tsp. SALT
    1/4 tsp. PEPPER
    1 cup dry BREAD CRUMBS
    1/4 cup VEGETABLE OIL

Preheat oven to 425 degrees. Rinse chicken breast halves; pat dry with paper towels.

Beat egg whites until frothy. Add milk, and beat again.

Combine flour, paprika, basil, salt, and pepper in large plastic food storage bag. Place bread crumbs in another bag. Dip breast halves, one or two at a time, in flour mixture, then in egg white mixture, then in crumbs.

Place oil in 15-1/4 x 10-1/4 x 3/4 inch broiler pan or other shallow pan. Place in oven for 3 or 4 minutes or until oil is hot, but not smoking. Add chicken breasts in single layer.

Bake for 20 minutes; turn chicken over; bake for 5 minutes.

A perfect meal with a tossed salad, Lemon Garlic Asparagus (see see page 174), and Banana Cream Pie(see page 235).

MAKES 8 SERVINGS
SERVING SIZE: 1 CHICKEN BREAST
CALORIES 240 • CHOL.: 65 MG. • FAT: 8 G. • SODIUM: 220 MG.

---

*=Dangerous to some • **=Consume with caution • See pages 19-22 for more information

Poultry Sausage Patties

Try serving these poultry burgers like hamburgers.

Quick and Easy

        3 Tbsp. MARGARINE
        1 lb. boneless uncooked CHICKEN BREAST (or TURKEY), coarsely ground
        1 cup fresh BREAD CRUMBS
        1 Tbsp. POULTRY SEASONING
        2 tsp. GROUND SAGE
        1/2 tsp. FENNEL SEED
        1/4 tsp. PEPPER
        1 tsp. BASIL LEAVES
        3 Tbsp. EGG SUBSTITUTE or 1 large EGG

Melt 2 tablespoons margarine; combine with chicken and bread crumbs in a bowl; set aside.

Crush spices together and mix with egg substitute; combine with chicken mixture. Shape into eight 3-inch round patties, using about 2 tablespoons of mixture for each patty.

Melt remaining margarine in a large skillet over medium heat. Cook patties 5 to 8 minutes on each side, until lightly browned and cooked through. Serve hot.

MICROWAVE: Prepare patties as above. Omit remaining tablespoon margarine. Place 4 patties in 9-inch microwave-proof pie plate. Microwave on medium (50% power) for 8 to 12 minutes, rotating a half turn after 1-1/2 minutes. Repeat with remaining patties.

Serve with Sweet Potatoes à l'Orange (see page 184) and Banana Snacking Cake (page 236).

MAKES 8 SERVINGS
SERVING SIZE: 1 PATTY
CALORIES: 121 • CHOL.: 33 MG. • FAT: 5 G. • SODIUM: 111 MG.

---

*=Dangerous to some • **=Consume with caution • See pages 19-22 for more information

Savory Lemon Chicken

There never seems to be any of this dish left over. Have you ever
noticed that it's the first one finished at a Chinese restaurant?

Prepare Ahead

Lemon juice**, Lemon **

NONSTICK COOKING SPRAY
2 whole CHICKEN BREASTS, split and skinned (about 1-1/2 lbs.)
1 can (10-3/4 oz.) CREAM OF CHICKEN SOUP
1 Tbsp. LEMON JUICE**
1/2 tsp. PAPRIKA
1/4 cup chopped SWEET RED PEPPERS
1 Tbsp. chopped fresh PARSLEY
4 LEMON SLICES** for garnish

Spray 10-inch skillet with cooking spray. Over medium heat, cook chicken 10 minutes or until browned on both sides.

In small bowl, combine soup, lemon juice, and paprika. Stir into skillet. Reduce heat to low. Cover; simmer 25 minutes, stirring occasionally.

Add red pepper and parsley. Cover; cook 10 minutes or until chicken is fork-tender, stirring occasionally. Serve sauce over chicken. Garnish with lemon slices.

Add Oriental Spinach (see page 178) and Parsley Potato Cakes (see page 179) to complement this dish.

TIP: To reduce sodium content, use low-sodium soup.

MAKES 4 SERVINGS
SERVING SIZE: 1/2 CHICKEN BREAST
CALORIES: 293 • CHOL.: 85MG. • FAT: 13 G. • SODIUM: 768 MG.

---

*=Dangerous to some • **=Consume with caution • See pages 19-22 for more information

Southwest Chicken

An easy-to-prepare dish of tender chicken.

Easy • Prepare Ahead

NONSTICK COOKING SPRAY
4 boneless CHICKEN BREASTS, skin removed
1 jar (12 oz.) CHUNKY SALSA (mild, medium, or hot)

Coat baking dish with cooking spray. Place chicken in baking dish; spread salsa evenly over chicken. Cover and marinate in refrigerator 1/2 hour, if possible. Preheat oven to 350 degrees. Bake 40 to 60 minutes.

MICROWAVE: Arrange chicken in microwave-safe baking dish; spread salsa evenly over chicken. Cover with waxed paper and marinate in refrigerator 1/2 hour if possible. Remove from refrigerator and place in microwave. Cook on medium (50% power) for 10 minutes. Turn dish or rearrange chicken and cook for 8 minutes more or until tender.

Jicama Salad (see page 70) goes well with this dish, with Caramel Custard (see page 239) to top off the meal.

MAKES 4 SERVINGS
SERVING SIZE: 1 CHICKEN BREAST
CALORIES: 199 • CHOL.: 77 MG. • FAT: 4 G. • SODIUM: 265 MG.

Spicy Orange Turkey

Another way of serving turkey so that it doesn't become boring.
Your taste buds will be pleased by this variation.

Quick and Easy

Onion powder**, Orange**, Orange juice**, Lemon juice**

12 oz. fully-cooked TURKEY BREAST, skinned

1/2 cup WATER

3 Tbsp. ORANGE JUICE CONCENTRATE**

1 Tbsp. LEMON JUICE**

1 tsp. CHILI POWDER

1/2 tsp. ONION POWDER**

4 tsp. CORNSTARCH

1 medium GREEN PEPPER, cut into 1-inch chunks

1 large ORANGE**, peeled and sliced crosswise

Cut turkey into 1/8-inch slices. Combine water, orange juice concentrate, lemon juice, chili powder, onion powder, and cornstarch in skillet. Heat on medium, stirring constantly until thickened. Layer turkey, green pepper, and orange slices in skillet. Bring to a boil; turn down heat. Cover; simmer 6 to 8 minutes. Place turkey in center of serving platter, and place orange slices and green pepper around edge. Stir sauce; pour small amount over turkey. Place remaining sauce in bowl to be used over turkey as desired.

MICROWAVE: Cut turkey into 1/8-inch slices; combine water, orange juice concentrate, lemon juice, chili powder, onion powder, and cornstarch in a microwave-safe baking dish. Cook 3 to 4 minutes on high or until thickened. Stir every minute. Layer turkey, green pepper, and orange slices in dish. Cook 6 to 8 minutes, turning dish every 2 minutes. Garnish and serve as above.

MAKES 4 SERVINGS

SERVING SIZE: 1/3 CUP

CALORIES: 241 • CHOL.: 68 MG. • FAT: 8 G. • SODIUM: 74 MG.

Stir-Fry Chicken and Broccoli

An Oriental way to prepare chicken; the combination of ingredients and aroma will have mouths watering throughout your home.

Quick

Green onions**

4 boneless, skinned whole CHICKEN BREASTS
or 8 thighs, skinned and boned

1/4 tsp. GROUND GINGER

1/4 tsp. PEPPER

4 tsp. VEGETABLE OIL

16-20 oz. frozen BROCCOLI, bits and pieces

1 cup sliced GREEN ONION**

1 cup CHICKEN BROTH, divided

1/2 tsp. SUGAR

SALT to taste

1 Tbsp. CORNSTARCH

Cut chicken into bite-sized pieces; sprinkle with ginger and pepper. Heat oil in large frying pan or wok over high heat. Add chicken and stir-fry 3 minutes or until brown; remove from pan and set aside. Add broccoli and onion; stir-fry 3 minutes. Mix 3/4 cup chicken broth with sugar and salt. Stir in vegetables; return chicken to pan. Reduce heat to medium-high; cover and cook 2 minutes. Mix cornstarch and remaining 1/4 cup chicken broth. Stir into pan and cook, stirring, for 1 minute. Remove from heat.

Glazed Apple Tart (see page 245) is a perfect finish for this meal.

MAKES 4 SERVINGS
SERVING SIZE: 1/2 CUP BROCCOLI AND 1 CHICKEN BREAST OR 2 THIGHS
CALORIES: 324 • CHOL.: 97 MG. • FAT: 15 G. • SODIUM: 286 MG.

Texas Style Duck

A unique entrée specialty.

Specialty

Onion**, Pecans**, Orange**

Stuffing:

> 1 cup diced CELERY
> 1 cup minced ONION**
> 1 cup coarsely chopped PECANS**
> 4 cups soft BREAD CRUMBS
> 1-1/2 tsp. SALT
> 1/2 cup EGG SUBSTITUTE, or 2 EGGS
> 1/2 cup MILK, scalded

Combine celery, onion, pecans, bread crumbs, salt; add to egg substitute. Mix well. Add scalded milk and blend.

MAKES 4-6 SERVINGS
SERVING SIZE: 1/2 CUP
CALORIES: 160 • CHOL. 0 • FAT: 2 G. • SODIUM: 479 MG.

Ducks:

> Two 2-1/2 lb. DUCKS
> 6 slices TURKEY BACON
> 1/2 cup CHILI SAUCE
> 1 cup CATSUP
> PARSLEY
> ORANGE SLICES**

Preheat oven to 500 degrees. Stuff ducks—both neck opening and between legs (vent)—with stuffing. Close both cavities by drawing the skin together, and stitch or skewer in place. Place 3 strips of bacon across the breast of each duck. Place on a rack in an uncovered roaster or baking pan. Roast for 15 minutes, then reduce heat to 350 degrees and roast until tender (allow 60 minutes per pound). A meat thermometer is helpful. (Temperature should reach 185 degrees.)

continued…

Remove bacon when it becomes brown. One-half hour before removing from oven, mix chili sauce and catsup together and pour over duck.

Arrange duck on a hot platter; garnish with parsley and orange slices.

Serve with a watercress-grapefruit section salad with Flavorful French Dressing (see page 82), Wild Rice Casserole (see page 186), Green Beans Delicious (see page 171), and Date-and-Nut Bread (see page 209).

MAKES 4-6 SERVINGS

SERVING SIZE: 3-1/2 OUNCES

WITH SKIN

CALORIES: 337 • CHOL.: 89 MG. • FAT: 28 G. • SODIUM: 357 MG.

WITHOUT SKIN

CALORIES: 201 • CHOL.: 84 MG. • FAT: 11 G. • SODIUM: 60 MG.

Turkey Quiche

An excellent way to serve leftover turkey.

Easy • Prepare Ahead

1 cup diced cooked TURKEY
1 9-inch SINGLE CRUST FLAKY PIE CRUST (see Desserts)
1 cup SKIM MILK
1 carton (8 oz.) EGG SUBSTITUTE, or 4 EGGS
1/4 cup minced fresh PARSLEY
2 Tbsp. diced PIMENTOS
1/2 tsp. GROUND SAGE
1/8 tsp. PEPPER

Preheat oven to 350 degrees. Spread turkey in bottom of unbaked pie crust shell. Combine skim milk, egg substitute, parsley, pimento, sage, and pepper; pour mixture over turkey. Bake for 45 to 50 minutes or until knife inserted in center comes out clean. Allow to stand 10 minutes. Cut into wedges and serve.

MAKES 6 SERVINGS
SERVING SIZE: 1/6 OF PIE
CALORIES: 255 • CHOL.: 18 MG. • FAT: 11 G. • SODIUM: 178 MG.

Turkey Chili

Cooking time is less than a half-hour for this hearty, nutritious and popular dish.

Quick and Easy • Prepare Ahead

Kidney beans*, Onion**

1 lb. GROUND TURKEY
1/4 cup DRIED ONION**
1/2 medium GREEN PEPPER, chopped
1/2 cup sliced CELERY
1/4 tsp. GARLIC POWDER
1 can (6 oz.) TOMATO PASTE
1 can (15-1/2 or 16 oz.) KIDNEY BEANS*, with liquid
1/2 tsp. SALT
1 can (12 oz.) TOMATO JUICE
1 tsp. GROUND CUMIN or CHILI POWDER
1 can (14-1/2 oz.) STEWED TOMATOES

Place ground turkey, onion, green pepper, and celery in large skillet. Cook on medium heat for 10 minutes, stirring and separating turkey as it cooks. Add remaining ingredients. Bring to a boil, turn down heat. Simmer 5 minutes, stirring occasionally.

MICROWAVE: Place turkey, onion, green pepper, and celery in large microwave-proof casserole. Cook for 6 minutes or until no longer pink, stirring and separating turkey every 2 minutes. Add remaining ingredients. Cover; cook 10 more minutes. Stir after 5 minutes.

Add Baked Apple Crumble (see page 234) or Carrot Cake (see page 240) for a great finish to this excellent meal.

MAKES 6 SERVINGS
SERVING SIZE: 1-1/4 CUPS
CALORIES: 296 • CHOL.: 47 MG. • FAT: 6 G. • SODIUM: 349 MG.

*=Dangerous to some • **=Consume with caution • See pages 19-22 for more information

Turkey Steak Diane

If you can't find fresh turkey breast steaks in the meat cuts, look for turkey (or chicken) tenders—the tenderloin muscle of poultry.

Quick and Easy

Green onion**

2 Tbsp. MARGARINE, divided
1 lb. (4) fresh TURKEY BREAST STEAKS, skinned
3 Tbsp. chopped GREEN ONION**
2 Tbsp. WHITE VINEGAR
1 Tbsp. WATER
1 tsp. SALT
2 tsp. finely chopped FRESH PARSLEY, or 1/2 tsp. DRIED PARSLEY

Melt 1 tablespoon margarine in skillet over medium heat. When margarine begins to bubble, add turkey; cook 3 minutes, then turn. Turn down heat to medium-low; cover, and cook 5 minutes more or until juices run clear. Melt remaining margarine in small saucepan. Add green onion; cook over medium heat and stir 2 to 3 minutes. Add vinegar, water, and salt; cook 2 minutes more. Serve over turkey steaks; sprinkle with parsley.

MICROWAVE: Melt 1 tablespoon margarine in microwave-safe dish on medium power; add turkey. Cover, cook 3 minutes, then turn turkey over. Cook 3 more minutes. Let stand covered 5 minutes or until juices run clear. Melt remaining margarine in small microwave-safe dish on high power. Add green onion; cook and stir 1 to 2 minutes. Add vinegar, water, and salt, and cook 1 to 2 minutes more. Serve over turkey steaks; sprinkle with parsley.

MAKES 4 SERVINGS
SERVING SIZE: 1 TURKEY STEAK
CALORIES: 199 • CHOL.: 65 MG. • FAT: 9 G. • SODIUM: 130 MG.

Fish Entrées

Baked Halibut

A delicious fish favorite—low in calories, salt, and fat but still high in good taste.

Quick and Easy

Onion**, Lemon or Lime juice**

1/4 tsp. THYME, crushed
1/8 tsp. each ROSEMARY, SALT and PEPPER
2 to 2-1/2 lb. HALIBUT
2 medium ONIONS**, thinly sliced or julienned
2 CARROTS, sliced or julienned
2 stalks CELERY, sliced or julienned
2 Tbsp. LEMON or LIME JUICE**
1 Tbsp. melted MARGARINE or BUTTER

Preheat oven to 450 degrees. Combine thyme, rosemary, salt, and pepper; season halibut with mixture. Place half of vegetables in baking dish; place halibut on vegetables. Top halibut with remaining vegetables; drizzle with lemon or lime juice and margarine. Bake, allowing about 10 minutes cooking time per inch of thickness measured at its thickest part, or until halibut flakes easily when tested with a fork.

Serve with Roasted Garlic Potatoes (see page 182), peas, and Lemon Love Notes (see page 247).

MAKES 6 SERVINGS
SERVING SIZE: 5 OUNCES
CALORIES: 254 • CHOL.: 50 G. • FAT: 10 G. • SODIUM: 222 MG.S

"Creamed" Tuna Over Toast

To save time, chicken soup may be substituted for the broth and flour.
Toasted bread or muffins afford texture contrast with the creamed tuna and peas.

Quick and Easy

1-1/2 cups CHICKEN BROTH, divided
3 Tbsp. FLOUR
1 can (6-1/2 oz.) WATER-PACKED TUNA, drained
2 cups FROZEN PEAS
chopped PARSLEY
6 slices BREAD or 6 ENGLISH MUFFIN halves

In saucepan, bring 1 cup of chicken broth to boil. In a bowl, combine the other 1/2 cup broth with 3 tablespoons flour. Mix until smooth. Add flour mixture to broth in saucepan; mix until smooth. Add tuna and peas, and simmer 5 minutes. Adjust seasoning to taste. Toast the bread or English muffins; ladle creamed tuna mixture over toast or muffins.

MAKES 6 SERVINGS
SERVING SIZE: 2/3 CUP SAUCE OVER BASE
CALORIES: 230 • CHOL.: 13 MG. • FAT: 2 G. • SODIUM: 619 MG.

Curried Shrimp and Rice

A one-dish meal that is a real winner (especially suitable for buffets) because it is equally good served with hot entrées or cold, as well as with salad.

Easy • Prepare Ahead

Vanilla extract*, Curry powder*

1 can (20 oz.) crushed PINEAPPLE packed in juice, undrained

2 tsp. CURRY POWDER*

1/2 tsp. SALT

1/2 tsp. VANILLA EXTRACT*

1/2 tsp. COCONUT EXTRACT

1 can (6 oz.) WATER CHESTNUTS, drained and sliced

3 cups (1 lb.) cooked SHRIMP

3 cups cooked BROWN RICE

Preheat oven to 325 degrees. Combine pineapple and its juice with the curry powder, salt, and extracts; mix well. Add water chestnuts, shrimp, and rice, and again mix well. Spoon into a casserole or baking dish and bake, uncovered, for 30 minutes.

MAKES 8 SERVINGS

SERVING SIZE: 1 CUP

CALORIES: 191 • CHOL.: 111 MG. • FAT: 1 G. • SODIUM: 278 MG.

Fillet of Sole Amandine

The freshness of the fish is all important for taste. Also important is not overcooking fish. Cook only until it has lost its translucent color and is still moist and juicy.

Quick and Easy

Almonds**, Scallions**, Lemon juice**

3 Tbsp. sliced ALMONDS**
I lb. fresh SOLE FILLETS
2 Tbsp. ALL-PURPOSE FLOUR
dash PEPPER
I Tbsp. MARGARINE
I Tbsp. sliced SCALLIONS**
I Tbsp. LEMON JUICE**

In large skillet, toast almonds over low heat. Remove from skillet; set aside.

Cut fillets in half lengthwise. Combine flour and pepper; coat fillets with mixture. Melt margarine in skillet over medium heat. Sauté fillets until golden, turning once, about 2 to 3 minutes on each side. Remove from skillet to a warm platter.

Return almonds to skillet with scallions; toss and stir until warm. Spoon over fillets and sprinkle with lemon juice. Garnish with parsley and lemon wedges, if desired. Serve immediately.

MAKES 4 SERVINGS
SERVING SIZE: 4 OUNCES
CALORIES: 170 • CHOL.: 54 MG. • FAT: 6 G. • SODIUM: 117 MG.

Fish Creole

These Neptune nibbles can be a healthy highlight of the week.
Fish may not be a "brain food," but it is certainly a smart choice.

Specialty

`Onion**`

1 pkg. (16 oz.) frozen COD FILLETS
1 Tbsp. MARGARINE
1-1/2 cups chopped ONIONS**
1/2 cup chopped GREEN PEPPER
2 CLOVES GARLIC, minced
4 medium ripe TOMATOES, peeled and coarsely chopped
2 Tbsp. chopped PARSLEY
2 tsp. PAPRIKA
1/2 tsp. SUGAR
1/8 tsp. GROUND RED PEPPER
1 BAY LEAF
1 Tbsp. CORNSTARCH
1 Tbsp. WATER
2 cups hot cooked RICE (prepared without added salt)

Partially thaw cod fillets, leaving in a block.

Melt margarine in a large saucepan; add onions, green pepper, and garlic. Sauté until tender, about 5 minutes. Add tomatoes, parsley, paprika, sugar, red pepper, and bay leaf, and bring to a boil. Reduce heat, cover, and simmer 30 minutes.

Cut partially thawed cod into 1-inch square pieces. Add to sauce; cook about 5 minutes, stirring occasionally, until fish flakes easily with a fork. Remove bay leaf. Blend together cornstarch and water; add to creole and cook, stirring until slightly thickened. Serve with rice.

MICROWAVE: in 2-quart microwave-proof casserole, melt margarine on high (100% power) for 1/2 to 1 minute. Add onions, green pepper, and garlic. Microwave on high for 3-1/2 to 4-1/2 minutes until onion is translucent, stirring after 1-1/2 minutes. Add tomatoes, parsley, paprika,
continued...

*=Dangerous to some • **=Consume with caution • See pages 19-22 for more information

sugar, red pepper, and bay leaf; cover. Microwave on high for 10 to 12 minutes, stirring after 5 minutes.

Cut partially thawed cod into 1-inch square pieces. Add to sauce; cover. Microwave on high for 1-1/2 to 2 minutes, stirring after 1 minute. Remove bay leaf. Blend cornstarch and water; add to creole. Cover, and microwave on high for 1 minute or until slightly thickened. Let stand covered 3 to 5 minutes before serving.

MAKES 4 SERVINGS
SERVING SIZE: 1 CUP
CALORIES: 293 • CHOL.: 49 MG. • FAT: 4 G. • SODIUM: 98 MG.

Fish 'n Veggie Bundles

Seafood is the 1990s slim-down favorite.
This recipe gives a feeling of "just-for-you" in these packets.

Quick and Easy

Mushrooms*, Green onion**

4 FLOUNDER FILLETS (about 1 lb.)
1/4 lb. MUSHROOMS*, thinly sliced
1/2 cup chopped RED PEPPER
1/4 cup sliced GREEN ONIONS**
1/4 tsp. DRIED BASIL
1/4 tsp. SALT
1/8 tsp. freshly ground PEPPER
4 tsp. MARGARINE

Preheat oven to 425 degrees. Cut 4 (12-inch) lengths of aluminum foil. Place one fillet at short end of each piece of foil. Divide mushrooms, red pepper, and green onions evenly over fillets. Sprinkle with basil, salt, and pepper. Top each fillet with 1 teaspoon margarine. Bring other end of foil over and tightly seal to form a packet. Place packets on ungreased cookie sheet. Bake 10 to 12 minutes or until fish is firm but moist.

MAKES 4 SERVINGS
SERVING SIZE: 1 BUNDLE
CALORIES: 150 • CHOL.: 55 MG. • FAT: 5 G. • SODIUM: 260 MG.

Pasta Primavera with Salmon

Quick and Easy • Prepare Ahead

Mushrooms*, Onion**, Lime or Lemon**

1-1/2 cups sliced MUSHROOMS*

2 tsp. instant minced or chopped ONION**

2 Tbsp. MARGARINE

1 Tbsp. FLOUR

1/8 tsp. crushed BASIL

1/8 tsp. crushed OREGANO

1/2 cup SKIM MILK

1 lb. SALMON, cooked and flaked,
   or 2 cans (6 oz. each) WATER-PACKED TUNA, drained

1 small YELLOW SQUASH or ZUCCHINI, sliced and cooked crisp-tender

1/2 cup frozen PEAS, thawed

1/2 cup diced TOMATO

1 tsp. PARSLEY FLAKES

8 oz. SPINACH FETTUCCINE or SPAGHETTI, cooked and drained

SALT and PEPPER to taste

LIME or LEMON wedges** for garnish

Sauté mushrooms and onion in margarine. Add flour, basil and oregano; cook and stir 1 minute. Gradually add milk; cook and stir until thickened. Add salmon, squash, peas, tomato and parsley. Heat thoroughly. Toss hot fettuccine with vegetable mixture. Season to taste with salt and pepper, and garnish with lime or lemon wedges.

MICROWAVE: Melt margarine in medium microwave-safe bowl. Mix in mushrooms and onion; cook 2 to 3 minutes, stirring after 1 minute. Add flour, basil, and oregano. Cook for 30 seconds; stir. Gradually add milk; cook about 2 to 3 minutes or until thickened. Stir every minute. Add salmon, squash, peas, tomato, and parsley; cook 4 to 5 minutes or until heated through. Toss hot fettuccine with vegetables; season to taste. Garnish with lime or lemon wedges.

MAKES 6 SERVINGS

SERVING SIZE: 1-1/2 CUPS

CALORIES: 271 • CHOL.: 68 MG. • FAT: 8 G. • SODIUM: 110 MG.

*=Dangerous to some • **=Consume with caution • See pages 19-22 for more information

Saucy Fish

An easy-to-prepare seafood dish that starts with frozen fillets!

Easy

Mayonnaise*, Yogurt**

1 lb. frozen COD FILLETS (nonbreaded)
1 Tbsp. DIJON MUSTARD
1/2 cup PLAIN NONFAT YOGURT**
1 Tbsp. REDUCED-CALORIE MAYONNAISE* (check label)
BLACK PEPPER to taste

Preheat oven to 350 degrees. Place fillets in baking dish. Mix remaining ingredients; pour mix over fillets. Bake for 25 to 35 minutes, or until fish flakes.

MICROWAVE: Arrange fillets in microwave-safe dish with thickest parts to the outside. Mix remaining ingredients; pour over fillets. Cover with vented plastic wrap. Microwave on high (100% power) for 3 minutes. Turn dish or move less cooked parts to outside of dish. Re-cover and microwave 3 to 5 more minutes, or until fish flakes.

Cajun Rice (see page 84) and Yellow Squash Fritters (see page 187) fit go well with this recipe, especially when you add Honey Walnut Cake (see page 246) or Banana Snacking Cake (see page 236) for that final treat.

MAKES 4 SERVINGS
SERVING SIZE: 4 OUNCES
CALORIES: 142 • CHOL.: 63 MG. • FAT: 3 G. • SODIUM: 160 MG.

---

*=Dangerous to some • **=Consume with caution • See pages 19-22 for more information

Shrimp Sauté with Dijon Mustard

When shrimp is on sale, try this universal favorite.

Quick and Easy

Lemon juice**

2 Tbsp. MARGARINE
1 lb. large SHRIMP, peeled, deveined and butterflied
1 CLOVE GARLIC, crushed
3 Tbsp. DIJON MUSTARD
2 Tbsp. chopped FRESH PARSLEY or 1-1/2 tsp. DRIED PARSLEY
1 Tbsp. LEMON JUICE**
1/4 tsp. DRIED TARRAGON LEAVES
cooked RICE

In large skillet, heat margarine over medium-high heat. Add shrimp and garlic to margarine, and sauté for 4 to 5 minutes or until shrimp are pink. Remove from heat; stir in mustard, parsley, lemon juice, and tarragon. Serve immediately over rice.

MICROWAVE: In shallow 2-quart microwave-safe dish, microwave margarine on high (100% power) for 30 seconds or until melted. Add shrimp and garlic; cover. Microwave on high for 4 to 5 minutes or until shrimp are pink and tender. Stir in mustard, parsley, lemon juice, and tarragon. Serve immediately over hot rice.

MAKES 4 SERVINGS
SERVING SIZE: 4 OUNCES
CALORIES: 143 • CHOL.: 161 MG. • FAT: 7 G. • SODIUM: 85 MG.

Sweet and Sour Fish

*Be sure the raisins, as well as all dried fruit, are soft and
not hard and dried; sometimes fermentation has already begun.*

Specialty

Raisins*, Onion**

1-1/2 cups WHITE VINEGAR

3/4 cup WATER

1/3 cup SUGAR

2 cups sliced ONIONS**

3/4 cup GOLDEN SEEDLESS RAISINS*

1-1/2 lbs. WHITEFISH FILLETS

2 Tbsp. MARGARINE

2 Tbsp. ALL-PURPOSE FLOUR

dash PEPPER

1/4 cup EGG SUBSTITUTE, or 1 EGG

In large saucepan, boil vinegar, water, and sugar for 10 minutes. Add onions and raisins; cook 10 minutes. Add whitefish fillets; cover and simmer for 10 to 12 minutes. Remove fish; set aside. Strain out and set aside onions and raisins; reserve 1-1/2 cups liquid.

In small saucepan, melt margarine over medium heat. Stir in flour and pepper; cook 1 minute. Stir in reserved liquid and egg substitute. Cook and stir until thickened, about 2 to 3 minutes.

Pour sauce over fish; garnish with onions and raisins. Serve hot or at room temperature. Rice is a good choice as an accompaniment.

MAKES 6 SERVINGS

SERVING SIZE: 1-1/2 CUPS

CALORIES: 322 • CHOL.: 68 MG. • FAT: 11 G. • SODIUM: 107 MG.

Tuna Noodle Supreme

A one-dish seafood entrée, with flavors that blend well—peas, tuna and noodles. If desired, substitute mushroom soup for the cornstarch and milk (does increase sodium content).

Easy

Mushrooms*, Onion**, Lemon juice**

1 Tbsp. MARGARINE
2 cups sliced MUSHROOMS*
1 large RED PEPPER, diced
1 medium ONION**, chopped
2 cups LOW-FAT MILK
2 Tbsp. CORNSTARCH
1/2 tsp. HOT PEPPER SAUCE
2 cans (6-1/2 oz. each) WATER-PACKED TUNA, drained and flaked
1 cup frozen PEAS, thawed
2 Tbsp. LEMON JUICE**
8 oz. medium EGG NOODLES, cooked and drained

In medium skillet melt margarine over medium-high heat. Add mushrooms, red pepper, and onion; sauté 4 to 5 minutes or until vegetables are tender. In small bowl combine milk, cornstarch, and hot pepper sauce until smooth. Stir into vegetable mixture. Stirring constantly, bring to a boil and boil 1 minute. Reduce heat to low. Add tuna and peas; heat through. Stir in lemon juice. Serve over noodles.

MAKES 6 SERVINGS
SERVING SIZE: 1-1/4 CUPS SAUCE AND NOODLES
CALORIES: 310 • CHOL.: 50 MG. • FAT: 5 G. • SODIUM: 270 MG.

*=Dangerous to some • **=Consume with caution • See pages 19-22 for more information

Whitefish Stew

Some cafeterias are serve a fish stew. Serve in bowls
over fluffy rice for a flavorful, completely balanced meal.

Quick and Easy

Onion**

1-1/2 lbs. COD, POLLOCK, or ROCKFISH FILLETS, defrosted and drained

2 Tbsp. VEGETABLE OIL

2 medium GREEN PEPPERS, chopped

2 CARROTS, thinly sliced

1 large ONION**, chopped

1 large CLOVE GARLIC, minced

1 can (28 oz.) TOMATOES

1 can (12 oz.) TOMATO JUICE

1 tsp. SUGAR

1 tsp. BASIL, crushed

1/2 cup WHITE VINEGAR or FISH STOCK

Cut fish into 1-inch chunks. Heat oil in large pot; sauté green peppers, carrots, onion, and garlic in oil until onion is tender. Add tomatoes, tomato juice, sugar, and basil. Bring to boil; simmer 10 minutes. Add vinegar and fish; simmer 8 minutes longer, or until fish flakes easily when tested with a fork.

MICROWAVE: Cut fish into 1-inch chunks. Mix with remaining ingredients except oil and vinegar. Place in microwave-safe baking dish; cover with plastic wrap. Microwave on high (100% power) for 3 to 4 minutes. Let stand, covered, 1 to 2 minutes. Stir, add vinegar, and cook for 3 to 5 minutes more or until fish flakes easily.

Finish your meal with Lemon Love Notes (see page 247).

MAKES 7 SERVINGS

SERVING SIZE: 1-1/4 CUPS

CALORIES: 179 • CHOL.: 52 MG. • FAT: 6 G. • SODIUM: 342 MG.

Side Dishes

Apple-Glazed Acorn Squash

*A delicious variation for acorn squash; low in calories,
and high in vitamin A's precursor, beta-carotene.*

Quick and Easy

1 medium ACORN SQUASH (about 1-1/2 lb.)
2 Tbsp. frozen APPLE JUICE CONCENTRATE, thawed
1/8 tsp. CINNAMON
1/8 tsp. GROUND GINGER

Pierce whole squash with a fork several times, and place on a paper towel in microwave oven. Microwave on high (100% power) 4 minutes.

Cut squash into 4 wedges; discard seeds and membrane. Place, cut sides up, in an 11 x 7 x 2-inch baking dish. Pierce flesh several times with a fork; set aside.

Combine juice concentrate, cinnamon and ginger. Stir well, and brush over squash. Cover with heavy-duty plastic wrap; microwave on high power 6 to 8 minutes or until tender, rotating dish a half-turn after 3 minutes.

MAKES 4 SERVINGS
SERVING SIZE: 1/4 SQUASH
CALORIES: 63 • CHOL.: 0 • FAT: 0.2 G. • SODIUM: 6 MG.

Austrian Cooked Cabbage

*Cabbage is an inexpensive source of vitamin C
and an anti-cancer, cruciferous vegetable.*

Quick and Easy

    NONSTICK COOKING SPRAY
    1/4 cup WHITE VINEGAR
    3 cups shredded RED CABBAGE
    1 tart APPLE, chopped
    1 tsp. CLOVES

Sauté cabbage until tender in a non-stick pan sprayed with cooking spray.
Add vinegar, apple, and cloves. Simmer until desired texture.

MAKES 2 SERVINGS
SERVING SIZE: 1 CUP
CALORIES: 90 • CHOL. 0 • FAT: 1 G. • SODIUM: 38 MG.

Baby Carrots with Dill

*A simple way to make carrots "gourmet." Chefs define "gourmet"
as interesting (not necessarily expensive, difficult to prepare, or foreign!).*

Quick and Easy

    1 lb. BABY CARROTS, scrubbed but not peeled
    2 Tbsp. FRESH DILL, chopped, or 1/2 tsp. DRIED DILL
    WATER

Steam baby carrots and dill in steamer or covered saucepan (use 1 inch
water) until tender. Serve hot or cold.

MAKES 4 SERVINGS
SERVING SIZE: 2/3 CUP
CALORIES: 42 • CHOL.: 0 • FAT: 0 • SODIUM: 47 MG.

*=Dangerous to some • **=Consume with caution • See pages 19-22 for more information

Cinnamon Apples

When an apple has lost its crispness, bake it, or
make this welcome addition to any meal, hot or cold.

Quick and Easy

Lemon juice**

1 medium tart APPLE, thinly sliced
2 tsp. LEMON JUICE**
1 tsp. MARGARINE
2 Tbsp. SUGAR (or sweetener to taste)
1/8 tsp. GROUND CINNAMON

Toss apple with lemon juice; set aside. Melt margarine in a nonstick skillet over medium heat. Add sugar and cinnamon; stir well. Add apple. Cook 7 minutes or until tender, stirring occasionally.

MAKES 2 SERVINGS
SERVING SIZE: 1/3 CUP
CALORIES: 106 • CHOL.: 0 • FAT: 2.1 G. • SODIUM: 23 MG.

Grilled Zucchini

Another great way to serve zucchini.

Easy

Lime juice**

    I small ZUCCHINI (about I lb.)
    2 Tbsp. OLIVE OIL
    I tsp. dried OREGANO
    I LIME**, juiced
    SALT and PEPPER to taste

Slice zucchini in half lengthwise. Rub with olive oil. Sprinkle with pepper and oregano; let rest for about 30 minutes.

Preheat broiler. Place zucchini on baking pan, cut sides up. Broil close to the heat until well browned. Remove from heat; sprinkle with lime juice. Season to taste.

MAKES 6 SERVINGS
SERVING SIZE: 1/2 CUP
CALORIES: 58 • CHOL.: 0 • FAT: 4 G. • SODIUM: 2 MG.

---

*=Dangerous to some • **=Consume with caution • See pages 19-22 for more information

Glazed Carrots

A beautiful, crunchy way to serve carrots. Remember that cornstarch or flour must be mixed with cold water (or fat) before adding to a hot mixture, and then brought to a boil to cook the starch.

Quick and Easy

Orange peel**, Walnuts**

1 lb. CARROTS, scraped and thickly sliced (about 3-1/2 cups)
WATER
1 Tbsp. MARGARINE
1/4 cup firmly packed LIGHT BROWN SUGAR
1 Tbsp. grated ORANGE PEEL**
2 Tbsp. cold WATER
1-1/2 tsp. CORNSTARCH
2 Tbsp. WALNUTS**, chopped

Cook carrots in small amount of unsalted water just until tender-crisp. Drain well.

Melt margarine in a large skillet; stir in brown sugar and orange peel. Cook until sugar melts and mixture thickens. Add water and cornstarch; blend until smooth. Add carrots, and cook over low heat for 10 minutes, stirring occasionally, until tender and glazed. Top with walnuts and serve.

MICROWAVE: In 1-quart microwave-safe casserole, cover and microwave carrots, margarine, and brown sugar on high (100% power) for 9 to 11 minutes, stirring after 5 minutes.

Blend 2 tablespoons cold water and 1-1/2 teaspoons cornstarch until smooth; stir into carrot mixture with orange peel and walnuts; cover. Microwave on high for 2 to 4 minutes or until thickened. Stir before serving.

MAKES 6 SERVINGS
SERVING SIZE: 2/3 CUP
CALORIES: 97 • CHOL.: 0 • FAT: 8 G. • SODIUM: 42 MG.

Green Beans Delicious

This recipe is really a winner; frozen green beans are also successful.
For guests, prepare the sautéed vegetables the day before and cook
the beans on the day of the party.

Quick and Easy • Prepare Ahead • Gourmet

Onion**

1 lb. (4 cups) GREEN BEANS
1/4 cup diced CELERY
1 tsp. chopped ONION**
1 tsp. minced GREEN PEPPER
2 Tbsp. OLIVE OIL
1 tsp. SUGAR
1/4 cup COTTAGE CHEESE
SALT to taste

Cook beans in boiling water (or steam or microwave), until tender; drain
if any water remains. Cook celery, onion, and green pepper in olive oil
until soft and yellow; add to hot beans. Add sugar and salt to taste. Heat.
Top with cottage cheese.

MAKES 6 SERVINGS
SERVING SIZE: 1/2 CUP
CALORIES: 82 • CHOL. 2 MG. • FAT: 5 G. • SODIUM: 42 MG.

Italian Steamed Artichokes

If you've never tried artichokes, try this low-calorie, easy dish.

Quick and Easy

1 large ARTICHOKE (about 1 lb.)
1 GARLIC CLOVE, sliced thin
1 BAY LEAF
1/4 tsp. CORIANDER SEEDS
1/2 tsp. DRIED OREGANO
1/2 tsp. DRIED BASIL

Snip the thorns off the artichoke leaves. Place the garlic slices inside the leaves throughout the artichoke. Put the artichoke into a medium-size saucepan. Add water to come halfway up the artichoke. Put the bay leaf in the water. Crush the coriander seeds, oregano, and basil together; sprinkle on top of the artichoke. Cook over medium heat for 30 minutes or until the leaves pull off easily.

MAKES 1 SERVING
SERVING SIZE: 1 ARTICHOKE
CALORIES: 44 • CHOL.: 0 • FAT: 0 • SODIUM: 30 MG.

Minted Citrus Carrots

The mint makes these carrots different. The sauce can also be served on hot, cooked carrots.

Quick and Easy • Prepare Ahead

Orange juice**, Lemon juice**

juice of 1 medium ORANGE**
juice of 1 medium LEMON**
1/4 cup freshly chopped MINT
1/8 tsp. PEPPER
3 large CARROTS, peeled and shredded

In small bowl, whisk juices, mint, and pepper together. Toss with shredded carrots and refrigerate. Serve cold.

MAKES 4 SERVINGS
SERVING SIZE: 1/2 CUP
CALORIES: 52 • CHOL.: 0 • FAT: 0 • SODIUM: 36 MG.

Lemon-Garlic Asparagus

A tasty method for preparing asparagus; use microwave if preferred.

Quick and Easy

Onion**, Lemon rind, Lemon juice**

- 1 CLOVE GARLIC, crushed
- 1/2 tsp. THYME
- 1/2 tsp. PEPPER
- 1 cup LOW-SODIUM CHICKEN BROTH (or use CHICKEN BOUILLON and water)
- 1 medium ONION**, sliced
- 1 tsp. grated LEMON RIND**
- 2 Tbsp. LEMON JUICE**
- 1 BAY LEAF
- 1 lb. fresh ASPARAGUS SPEARS

Combine all of the ingredients except asparagus in a saucepan. Cover and simmer 15 minutes, then remove bay leaf. Wash asparagus in cold water. Break off tough ends. Add asparagus to the saucepan. Cover and simmer just until asparagus is tender.

MAKES 4 SERVINGS
SERVING SIZE: 1/2 CUP
CALORIES: 42 • CHOL. : 0 • FAT: 0 • SODIUM: 4 MG.

Lemon-Herb Twice Baked Potatoes

These popular stuffed baked potatoes have become almost a staple in American diets. They can be prepared ahead of time and successfully reheated.

Prepare Ahead

Onion**, Lemon peel**

6 small BAKING POTATOES (4 to 6 oz. each)
1/3 cup chopped ONION**
I CLOVE GARLIC, minced
2 Tbsp. MARGARINE
1/2 cup hot SKIM MILK
I tsp. grated LEMON PEEL**
1/8 tsp. GROUND WHITE PEPPER
I Tbsp. chopped FRESH DILL or I tsp. DILL WEED
I Tbsp. finely chopped PARSLEY
PAPRIKA

Bake potatoes at 400 degrees until done, about 45 minutes. Let stand at room temperature until cool enough to handle. Meanwhile, sauté onion and garlic in margarine until tender; set aside. Cut a slice from the top of each potato; scoop out the insides, being careful not to break skins. Mash potato insides; beat in prepared onion mixture, hot skim milk, lemon peel ,and pepper. Mix in dill and parsley. Place potato skins in a baking dish. Pile mashed potato mixture into skins; sprinkle with paprika. Bake at 400 degrees for 30 minutes or until light brown.

MICROWAVE: Pierce potatoes with fork. Place 1 inch apart on paper toweling in microwave oven. Microwave on high (100% power) for 15 to 17 minutes or until tender, turning over and rearranging after 10 minutes. In 1-quart microwave-safe glass measure, melt margarine on high for 1/2 to 1 minute. Add onion and garlic. Microwave on high for 1 minute. Prepare filling and stuff potatoes as above. Arrange in a 9-inch microwave-proof pie plate. Microwave on high for 4 to 5 minutes or until heated through, rearranging after 2 minutes.

MAKES 6 SERVINGS
SERVING SIZE: I STUFFED POTATO
CALORIES: 150 • CHOL: 0 • FAT: 4 G. • SODIUM: 53 MG.

*=Dangerous to some • **=Consume with caution • See pages 19-22 for more information

Mexican Corn

A colorful way to serve frozen corn or off-the-cob fresh corn.

Quick and Easy

2 Tbsp. MARGARINE
1 pkg. (10 oz.) frozen WHOLE KERNEL GOLDEN CORN
1/2 cup chopped GREEN PEPPER
1 CLOVE GARLIC, crushed
dash BLACK PEPPER
1 Tbsp. PIMENTO pieces or chopped RED BELL PEPPERS
WARM WATER

Melt margarine in a saucepan over medium heat. Stir in corn, green pepper, garlic, and black pepper. Cover and simmer for 10 minutes, stirring occasionally. Mix in pimento and continue cooking 2 minutes or until corn is tender. If necessary, stir in a little warm water to prevent sticking. Serve hot.

MICROWAVE: In a 1-1/2 quart microwave-safe casserole, microwave margarine on high (100% power) for 40 to 45 seconds. Add corn, green pepper, garlic, black pepper, and pimento. Cover; microwave on high for 4 to 5 minutes, stirring once. Stir before serving.

MAKES 4 SERVINGS
SERVING SIZE: 1/2 CUP
CALORIES: 117 • CHOL.: 0 • FAT: 6 G. • SODIUM: 51 MG.

New Potatoes in Lemon Parsley Sauce

The lemon peel and chopped parsley add interest to the wonderful flavor of new potatoes.

Quick and Easy

Lemon peel**, Lemon juice**

4 whole NEW POTATOES (about 1/2 lb.)
BOILING WATER
1 Tbsp. MARGARINE
1/2 tsp. grated LEMON PEEL**
1 Tbsp. LEMON JUICE**
1 Tbsp. chopped PARSLEY

Cook potatoes in boiling water for 15 to 20 minutes or until tender. Drain, peel, and quarter (if desired).

Melt margarine in saucepan over low heat; mix in lemon peel, lemon juice, and parsley. Add potatoes and cook over medium heat, turning frequently, until hot and coated with margarine.

MICROWAVE: In covered 1-quart microwave-safe casserole, microwave potatoes and 1/4 cup water on high (100% power) for 5 to 7 minutes. Drain, peel, and quarter potatoes, if desired. In same dish, microwave margarine on high for 30 seconds. Add lemon peel, lemon juice, parsley, and potatoes. Microwave on high for 30 seconds. Toss potatoes to coat with margarine before serving.

MAKES 2 SERVINGS
SERVING SIZE: 2 NEW POTATOES (4 OUNCES)
CALORIES: 142 • CHOL.: 0 • FAT: 6 G. • SODIUM: 57 MG.

*=Dangerous to some • **=Consume with caution • See pages 19-22 for more information

Oriental Spinach

Quick and Easy

1 tsp. WHITE VINEGAR
1/2 tsp. SOY SAUCE**
1/4 tsp. POWDERED GINGER
1-1/2 Tbsp. WATER
SWEETENER to taste
NONSTICK COOKING SPRAY
1 CLOVE GARLIC, crushed
1 lb. FRESH SPINACH, washed and drained (tough portions of stem removed), large leaves cut in pieces

Mix vinegar, soy sauce, ginger, water, and sweetener in a bowl and set aside. Spray wok or frying pan with cooking spray. Heat; add garlic. Stir-fry 10 seconds. Add spinach and stir-fry 1 minute or until wilted. Add sauce mixture; stir and serve.

MAKES 3 SERVINGS
SERVING SIZE: 1/2 CUP
CALORIES: 41 • CHOL.: 0 • FAT: 0.5 G. • SODIUM: 165 MG.

---

*=Dangerous to some • **=Consume with caution • See pages 19-22 for more information

Parsley Potato Cakes

Everyone seems to like potato patties.

Quick and Easy

> 4 cups MASHED POTATOES, cold
> 2 Tbsp. OLIVE OIL
> 1/4 cup PARSLEY, chopped
> 1/2 tsp. MUSTARD POWDER
> 1/2 tsp. GARLIC POWDER
> FLOUR, as needed
> NONSTICK COOKING SPRAY

Combine potatoes, oil, parsley, mustard powder, and garlic powder in large bowl. Mix well; form mixture into patties. Dip patties in flour; shake off excess. Spray cool pan with cooking spray in frying pan; place pan over medium heat. Add patties; cook until golden brown on both sides.

MAKES 6 SERVINGS
SERVING SIZE: ONE 2/3 CUP PATTY
CALORIES: 252 • CHOL.: 18 MG. • FAT: 16 G. • SODIUM: 474 MG.

Peas Superb

A delicious way to serve peas; frozen peas also work well, but shorten the cooking time. If microwaving, stir frozen peas into mushroom mixture.

Quick and Easy

Mushrooms*, Onion**

2-1/2 cups FRESH PEAS (about 2 lbs., unshelled)
BOILING WATER
1 Tbsp. MARGARINE
1 cup sliced fresh MUSHROOMS*
2 Tbsp. chopped ONION**

Cook peas in a small amount of boiling water until tender. Melt margarine in large skillet. Add mushrooms and onion, and sauté until tender; add peas and cook until heated through. Serve immediately.

MICROWAVE: In 1-quart microwave-safe bowl, cover and microwave peas and 1/4 cup water on high (100% power) for 7 to 8 minutes, stirring after 4 minutes. Drain; set aside.

In 1-quart microwave-proof casserole, microwave margarine on high for 30 seconds; stir in mushrooms and onions. Microwave on high for 1 minute. Stir in peas; microwave on high for 2 to 3 minutes, stirring after 1-1/2 minutes. Stir before serving.

MAKES 5 SERVINGS
SERVING SIZE: 1/2 CUP
CALORIES: 88 • CHOL.: 0 • FAT: 3 G. • SODIUM: 24 MG.

*=Dangerous to some • **=Consume with caution • See pages 19-22 for more information

Potato Pancakes

Potato pancakes made with raw potatoes are more flavorful than those made with mashed potatoes. White pepper not only looks more attractive with white foods, but tastes different, too.

Quick and Easy

`Onion**`

1/2 cup EGG SUBSTITUTE, or 2 EGGS
3 cups cubed raw POTATOES
1/2 cup coarsely chopped ONION**
1/4 cup ALL-PURPOSE FLOUR
1/8 tsp. GROUND WHITE PEPPER
2 Tbsp. MARGARINE
APPLESAUCE (optional)

Place egg substitute in blender container; add potatoes, onion, flour, and pepper. Blend until potatoes are well grated and the mixture is evenly rough in consistency.

Melt 1 teaspoon margarine on hot griddle for every 2 pancakes. For each pancake, pour 1/4 cup batter onto hot griddle. Fry on both sides until well browned, about 3 minutes per side. Serve hot with applesauce, if desired.

MAKES 1 DOZEN PANCAKES, 6 SERVINGS
SERVING SIZE: 2 SMALL PANCAKES
CALORIES: 125 • CHOL.: 0 • FAT: 4 G. • SODIUM: 63 MG.

*=Dangerous to some • **=Consume with caution • See pages 19-22 for more information

Roasted Garlic Potatoes

These crusty potatoes, with their crunchy surface and tender interior, are a favorite of many. Potatoes also are a good source of vitamin C.

Easy

Onion**

1/4 cup OLIVE OIL
1 medium ONION**, sliced
2 Tbsp. GARLIC, minced
1 lb. RED POTATOES

Preheat oven to 375 degrees. Heat oil in skillet. Add onions and garlic. Sauté until just golden. Cut potatoes into wedges; add to skillet. Sauté until golden brown and well coated. Transfer to baking pan; bake until dark golden brown and fork tender, about 20 minutes.

MAKES 6 SERVINGS
SERVING SIZE: 1/2 CUP
CALORIES: 150 • CHOL.: 0 • FAT: 9 G. • SODIUM: 7 MG.

Steamed Spring Asparagus

Serve with creamed tuna or chicken for lunch or supper.

Quick and Easy

1/4 cup SUGAR
1 lb. SPRING ASPARAGUS, trimmed
1 quart BOILING WATER
1/2 stick BUTTER (1/4 cup)
SALT and PEPPER to taste

Heat heavy saucepan. Add sugar; stir just until melted. Add asparagus and boiling water. Cover pan; boil hard for 5 minutes. Drain. Add butter to asparagus; stir just until well coated and hot. Season to taste.

MAKES 6 SERVINGS
SERVING SIZE: 1/2 CUP
CALORIES: 94 • CHOL.: 22 MG. • FAT: 8 G. • SODIUM: 83 MG.

Sweet Potatoes à l'Orange

Quick and Easy

Dried apricots*, Orange**

2 lbs. SWEET POTATOES, cooked, or 2 pounds canned SWEET POTATOES
2 Tbsp. MARGARINE, melted
1/2 tsp. GROUND CINNAMON
16 DRIED APRICOT halves*
SWEETENER to taste
Fresh ORANGE SLICES**, cut into half circles

Preheat oven to 425 degrees. Arrange the sweet potatoes in a shallow baking dish. Combine the margarine and cinnamon. Pour over potatoes. Arrange the apricot halves on top. Cover the dish and bake for about 15 minutes. Add sweetener, if desired. Garnish with orange slices, and serve.

MAKES 8 SERVINGS
SERVING SIZE: 2/3 CUP
CALORIES: 185 • CHOL.: 0 • FAT: 7 G. • SODIUM: 79 MG.

Vegetable Mélange

*Save a few of these vegetables from your raw vegetable
purchases for a colorful combination of flavors.*

Quick and Easy

Onion**

1 small ZUCCHINI, shredded
1 small YELLOW SQUASH, shredded
2 CARROTS, shredded
1 small ONION**, sliced thin
2 Tbsp. WATER
2 tsp. MARGARINE

Combine the zucchini, yellow squash, carrots, onion, and water in a skillet. Cover and cook over medium heat for 4 to 5 minutes, or until vegetables are tender. Add margarine. Sauté uncovered until all moisture has evaporated. Serve immediately.

MAKES 2 SERVINGS
SERVING SIZE: 1/2 CUP
CALORIES: 94 • CHOL.: 0 • FAT: 4 G. • SODIUM: 83 MG.

Wild Rice Casserole

A great way to serve crunchy rice. Can be prepared the day before and reheated for a party. Delicious served with poultry. All brown rice works fine, too.

Prepare Ahead • Gourmet

Mushrooms*, Onion**

1/2 cup WILD RICE
1/2 cup BROWN RICE
1 cup WATER
1 box (4 oz.) MUSHROOMS* cut up, or 1 small can MUSHROOMS*
1 large ONION**, chopped
1 cup MEDIUM WHITE SAUCE, or 1 cup undiluted MUSHROOM SOUP*
NONSTICK COOKING SPRAY

Clean wild rice by putting it in a bowl of water, picking out hulls, etc.; drain. Cook all rice with the 1 cup of water, at low temperature, in tightly covered pan for about 1/2 hour. Don't let it get mushy.

In the meantime, spray skillet with cooking spray, and brown mushroom pieces and onion until slightly cooked, but still crunchy.

Stir white sauce or mushroom soup, rice, and onion-mushroom mixture together with a fork, only until lightly combined. Place in greased casserole to be baked now or later. Bake 25 minutes at 350 degrees.

MAKES 6 SERVINGS
SERVING SIZE: 2/3 CUP
CALORIES: 90 • CHOL.: 0 • FAT: 1 G. • SODIUM: 400 MG.

*=Dangerous to some • **=Consume with caution • See pages 19-22 for more information

Yellow Squash Fritters

Always save (or drink) the drained water from vegetables.
This liquid has much of the water-soluble vitamins.

Quick and Easy

`Onion**`

1 cup steamed, diced YELLOW SQUASH, well drained
1 EGG, or 1/4 cup EGG SUBSTITUTE
1 slice BREAD, crumbled
1 tsp. PARSLEY FLAKES
1 tsp. DRIED ONION FLAKES**
NONSTICK COOKING SPRAY

In blender combine all ingredients and blend just until squash is finely chopped. Drop by tablespoons onto griddle sprayed with cooking spray. Cook over moderate heat until browned on bottom. Turn and cook until top is browned.

MAKES 1 SERVING
SERVING SIZE: 1 FRITTER
CALORIES: 182 • CHOL.: 0 MG. • FAT: 2 G. • SODIUM: 80 MG.

Zucchini Sauté

A nice change from "just zucchini."

Quick and Easy

Mushrooms*

1 Tbsp. MARGARINE
3 medium ZUCCHINI, thinly sliced
1 small GREEN PEPPER, coarsely chopped
2 CLOVES GARLIC, minced
1 cup sliced fresh MUSHROOMS*
1/8 tsp. BLACK PEPPER

Melt margarine in large skillet over medium heat. Add zucchini, green pepper, and garlic. Sauté until zucchini is tender and crisp, about 5 minutes. Add mushrooms and pepper; cook and stir about 5 minutes more until vegetables are tender but firm.

MAKES 8 SERVINGS
SERVING SIZE: 1/2 CUP
CALORIES: 27 • CHOL.: 0 • FAT: 2 G. • SODIUM: 14 MG.

Sauces & Toppings

Pizza Party Base

*Everyone will be impressed that you can make your own pizza base.
Biscuit dough can substitute effectively, too—rolled to 1/8-inch thickness
—because it rises so much.*

Prepare Ahead

2-3/4 to 3-1/4 cups ALL-PURPOSE FLOUR, divided
1 Tbsp. SUGAR
1 pkg. ACTIVE DRY YEAST
1/4 cup MARGARINE
1 cup WATER
2 cups LOW-SODIUM TOMATO JUICE
3/4 cup (6 cubes) frozen LOW-SODIUM TOMATO BASE (see page 195)
   or TOMATO FRESH SALSA (see page 194)
1 tsp. OREGANO LEAVES
1/2 tsp. crushed fresh GARLIC
1/8 tsp. PEPPER

Mix 1 cup flour, sugar, and undissolved yeast. Heat margarine and water in a saucepan until very warm (120 to 130 degrees). Margarine does not need to melt. Gradually add to dry ingredients and beat 2 minutes with electric mixer at medium speed, scraping bowl occasionally; add 1/2 cup flour. Beat at high speed 2 minutes, scraping bowl occasionally.

Stir in enough additional flour to make a stiff dough. Turn out onto a floured board; knead until smooth and elastic, about 4 to 5 minutes. Place in a greased bowl, turning to grease top. Cover; let rise in a warm draft-free place until doubled in size, about 1 hour.

Combine tomato juice, tomato base, oregano, garlic, and pepper in a medium saucepan. Bring to a boil over medium-high heat, stirring occasionally. Reduce heat to low and simmer until reduced to 1-1/2 cups.

Punch dough down; divide in half. Shape each half into a ball; cover and let stand 10 minutes. Roll and stretch each half to a 14-inch circle. Place in 2 greased 14-inch pizza pans, forming a standing rim of dough around edges.

    continued...

---

*=Dangerous to some • **=Consume with caution • See pages 19-22 for more information

Spread half of prepared tomato sauce over each crust and top pies with either Vegetable Topping (see page 193) or Beef and Zucchini Topping (see next page). Bake at 375 degrees for 20 to 25 minutes or until done.

NOTE: If desired, pizza crust can be prebaked at 375 degrees for 7 minutes, then frozen. When ready to use, defrost crust; top and bake as directed above.

MAKES 2 (14-INCH) PIZZAS, 8 SLICES PER PIE
NUTRITIONAL VALUE INCLUDED IN RECIPES USING PIZZA CRUST

Beef and Zucchini Topping

Vary a pizza with this different topping; also can be used on stuffed baked potatoes or tortillas.

Quick and Easy

1 Tbsp. MARGARINE
1 cup sliced ZUCCHINI
1/4 lb. lean GROUND BEEF

Melt margarine in skillet over medium heat. Sauté sliced zucchini until tender crisp, about 2 to 3 minutes. Remove from pan. Crumble and brown ground beef in skillet over medium heat. Remove from skillet and drain well.

Arrange beef and zucchini on pizza crust and bake as directed (see Pizza Party Base, page 190).

MAKES 8 SERVINGS ON ONE 14-INCH PIZZA CRUST
SERVING SIZE: 1/8 PIZZA
CALORIES: 174 • CHOL.: 9 MG. • FAT: 6 G. • SODIUM: 97 MG.

Vegetable Topping
Another topping for pizza.

Quick and Easy

Mushrooms*, Onion**

1 Tbsp. MARGARINE
2 cups sliced MUSHROOMS*
3/4 cup thinly sliced GREEN PEPPER strips
3/4 cup thinly sliced ONION**

Melt margarine in skillet over medium heat. Sauté sliced mushrooms until slightly golden. Remove from heat. Toss in green pepper strips and sliced onion. Arrange topping on a 14-inch pizza crust and bake as directed (see Pizza Party Base, page 190).

MAKES 8 SERVINGS ON 14-INCH PIZZA CRUST
SERVING SIZE: 1/8 PIZZA
CALORIES: 165 • CHOL.: 5 MG. • FAT: 5 G. • SODIUM: 94 MG.

Tomato Fresh Salsa

This salsa has many uses; try it over eggs or as a dip with tortilla or corn chips.

Prepare Ahead

Onion**, Lemon juice**

3-1/2 cups (28 oz. can) CRUSHED TOMATOES
1/2 cup (4 oz.) diced GREEN CHILES
1/2 cup sliced GREEN ONIONS**, tops included
1/3 cup fresh LEMON JUICE**
2 Tbsp. finely chopped fresh CILANTRO or PARSLEY
2 tsp. DRIED OREGANO LEAVES, crushed
1-1/2 tsp. GARLIC SALT
1/2 tsp. GROUND CUMIN
1/4 tsp. RED PEPPER FLAKES (optional)

In large bowl, combine all ingredients. Mix well. Cover and refrigerate for 4 hours to allow flavors to blend.

TIP: Baked tortilla chips are lower in fat than fried chips.

MAKES 4-1/2 CUPS SALSA
SERVING SIZE: 1 TABLESPOON
CALORIES: 14 • CHOL.: 0 • FAT: 0 • SODIUM: 262 MG.

Low-Sodium Tomato Base

This on-hand tomato base adds its own special flavor to every dish that includes it.

Prepare Ahead

Onion**

5 lbs. ripe TOMATOES, coarsely chopped
1 cup chopped ONIONS**
1 cup grated CARROTS
1 cup minced RED PEPPER

Combine all ingredients in large heavy pan. Cover; cook over medium-high heat, stirring occasionally, until tomatoes are a liquid and pulp mixture, about 30 minutes. Uncover; cook over medium heat, stirring occasionally, until thickened and reduced by half, about 3-1/2 to 4 hours. Put mixture through a sieve to remove skins and seeds.

Place strained mixture in a medium saucepan. Partially cover and cook over medium heat until very thick, making about 3 cups. Cool.

Measure 2 tablespoons tomato base into individual ice cube tray sections. Freeze until firm. Remove from trays and store in a plastic bag or tightly closed container. Use as directed in recipes.

MAKES 3 CUPS (24 CUBES)
SERVING SIZE: 1 CUBE (2 TABLESPOONS)
CALORIES: 23 • CHOL.: 0 • FAT: 0 • SODIUM: 9 MG.

Easy Tomato Sauce

A marinara-type spaghetti sauce—the type Italian wives rushed to make when they first saw their sailor-husbands' ships appear homeward bound on the horizon.

Quick and Easy

Onion**

2 tsp. OLIVE OIL
1/2 cup finely chopped ONION**
2 CLOVES GARLIC, minced
2 cans (28 oz.) ITALIAN TOMATOES, undrained and chopped
2 tsp. minced FRESH OREGANO
1/8 to 1/4 tsp. PEPPER
1/4 cup chopped FRESH BASIL

Heat oil in a large skillet over medium-low heat until hot. Add onion, and sauté until tender. Add garlic; sauté 1 minute. Stir in tomatoes, and bring to a boil. Add remaining ingredients; stir well. Reduce heat to medium-low and cook, uncovered, until thickened, stirring frequently. Serve over cooked pasta.

VARIATION: Fiery Tomato and Red Pepper Sauce: add 1/4 teaspoon crushed red pepper to basil, oregano, and black pepper.

MAKES 4 CUPS
SERVING SIZE: 1/2 CUP
CALORIES: 56 • CHOL.: 0 • FAT: 1.6 G. • SODIUM: 324 MG.

Classic Iowa Barbecue Sauce

*A barbecue sauce that can be used on any meat, fish, or poultry.
The orange juice is the mystery ingredient.*

Quick and Easy

Orange juice**

1/2 cup CATSUP
1 CLOVE GARLIC, minced, or 1/4 tsp. GARLIC POWDER
1 Tbsp. ORANGE JUICE CONCENTRATE**
2 Tbsp. PREPARED MUSTARD
1 Tbsp. WHITE VINEGAR

Combine all ingredients. Spread over meat 4 minutes prior to removing from grill. Grill on one side for 2 minutes. Turn meat, coat the other side, and grill for an additional 2 minutes.

MAKES 2/3 CUP SAUCE
SERVING SIZE: 1 TABLESPOON
CALORIES: 40 • CHOL.: 0 • FAT: 1 G. • SODIUM: 255 MG.

*=Dangerous to some • **=Consume with caution • See pages 19-22 for more information

Green Onion Potato Topping

Quick and Easy

Mayonnaise*, Green onions**

1 cup cholesterol-free REDUCED-CALORIE MAYONNAISE* (check label)
1/4 cup sliced GREEN ONIONS**

Combine ingredients in a small bowl. Serve over baked potato.

MAKES 1 CUP
SERVING SIZE: 1 TABLESPOON
CALORIES: 50 • CHOL.: 0 • FAT: 3 G. • SODIUM: 80 MG.

Tomato and Mushroom Sauce

*Another spaghetti sauce to prepare ahead of time. Add a pinch of sugar
or sweetener to taste, as your grandmother used to, for added flavor.*

Prepare Ahead

Mushrooms*, Onion**

2 tsp. OLIVE OIL
1/2 cup finely chopped ONION**
2 CLOVES GARLIC, minced
2 cups chopped fresh MUSHROOMS*
2 cans (28 oz. each) ITALIAN TOMATOES, undrained and chopped
2 tsp. minced fresh OREGANO
1/8 to 1/4 tsp. PEPPER
1/4 cup chopped FRESH BASIL

Heat oil in a large skillet over medium-low heat until hot. Add onion, and
sauté until tender. Add garlic; sauté 1 minute. Add mushrooms to sautéed
onion mixture. Stir in tomatoes and bring to a boil. Add remaining ingredients and stir well. Reduce heat to medium-low and cook, uncovered,
1-1/2 hours or until thickened, stirring frequently.

MAKES 4 CUPS
SERVING SIZE: 1/2 CUP
CALORIES: 61 • CHOL.: 0 • FAT: 1.7 G. • SODIUM: 325 MG.

---

*=Dangerous to some • **=Consume with caution • See pages 19-22 for more information

Sauce Dijonnaise

Change the taste of plain vegetables with this sauce.

Quick and Easy

Lemon juice**

1/2 cup light, regular, or unsalted MARGARINE
1 Tbsp. LEMON JUICE**
1 Tbsp. DIJON MUSTARD
1/2 tsp. TARRAGON LEAVES

Melt margarine in small saucepan over medium heat. Whisk in lemon juice, mustard, and tarragon. Serve over hot cooked vegetables.

MAKES ABOUT 2/3 CUP

SERVING SIZE: 1 TABLESPOON

REGULAR MARGARINE

CALORIES: 82 • CHOL.: 0 • FAT: 9 G. • SODIUM: 121 MG.

UNSALTED MARGARINE

CALORIES: 82 • CHOL.: 0 • FAT: 9 G. • SODIUM: 45 MG.

LIGHT SPREAD

CALORIES: 42 • CHOL.: 0 • FAT: 5 G. • SODIUM: 125 MG.

Skinny-Dip Tartar Sauce

This low-cal tartar sauce will spice up any seafood entrée.

Quick and Easy

Yogurt**, Onion**

3/4 cup LOW-FAT COTTAGE CHEESE
1/4 cup PLAIN NONFAT YOGURT**
1 Tbsp. minced FRESH PARSLEY
1 Tbsp. chopped ONION**
2 Tbsp. grated CUCUMBER
1 tsp. CELERY FLAKES
1/2 tsp. CAPERS, or to taste

Blend cottage cheese in blender until smooth. Mix in all other ingredients and refrigerate. Use within 2 days.

MAKES 1-1/4 CUPS
SERVING SIZE: 1 TABLESPOON
CALORIES: 12 • CHOL.: 1 MG. • FAT: TRACE • SODIUM: 25 MG.

Vegetable Relish

This is the relish often seen in buffet or cafeteria serving lines.

Prepare Ahead

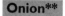

1 cup shredded CARROTS
1 cup chopped CUCUMBERS
1/2 cup chopped RED PEPPER
1/2 cup chopped GREEN PEPPER
1/4 cup finely chopped RED ONION**
3 Tbsp. WHITE VINEGAR
1 tsp. SUGAR
1/4 tsp. SALT
1 Tbsp. VEGETABLE OIL

Combine carrot, cucumber, peppers, and onion in a medium bowl. Set aside. Mix vinegar, sugar, and salt together. Add oil and whisk thoroughly. Pour over vegetables and toss to coat. Cover and refrigerate for at least 1 hour before serving.

MAKES 4 SERVINGS
SERVING SIZE: 3/4 CUP
CALORIES: 84 • CHOL.: 0 • FAT: 4 G. • SODIUM: 162 MG.

Festive Cranberry Sauce

Turkey, especially, seems more festive with cranberry sauce, and this one is tasty, yet different.

Quick and Easy • Prepare Ahead

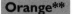

2 cups fresh CRANBERRIES
1 ORANGE**, peeled and chopped
1 cup frozen unsweetened STRAWBERRIES, defrosted
1 Tbsp. ARTIFICIAL SWEETENER
1/4 cup WATER

Put cranberries, orange, and water in medium saucepan. Simmer until cranberry skins burst, approximately 10 to 15 minutes. Remove from heat. Add sweetener to taste and strawberries. Chill and serve.

MAKES 4 SERVINGS
SERVING SIZE: 1/2 CUP
CALORIES: 63 • CHOL.: 0 • FAT: 0 • SODIUM: 1 MG.

Pear Butter

This treat is a great topping for toast or ice cream;
it even tastes good with meat dishes.

Prepare Ahead • Gourmet

Vanilla extract*, Lemon juice**

3-1/2 lb. PEARS, peeled and quartered (8 pears)
1/3 cup LEMON JUICE** (juice from 2 lemons)
1/2 cup MARGARINE
2-1/2 tsp. VANILLA EXTRACT*
4 tsp. granulated SUGAR SUBSTITUTE

Mix pears and lemon juice in a saucepan. Bring to a boil. Cook covered over very low heat for 15 minutes, or until pears are tender. Drain well and reserve juice.

In another pan, bring juice to a boil. Simmer until reduced to 1/4 cup. Blend pears in food processor or blender. Add hot juice, margarine (if using a stick, slice into sections), and vanilla. Blend until margarine is dissolved into pear mixture. Cool. Stir in sweetener. Pour pear butter in freezer bags or plastic freezer containers and refrigerate. (Pear butter will stay fresh in the refrigerator for about one week; freeze the extra pear butter be used later.)

MAKES 6 CUPS
SERVING SIZE: 1 TABLESPOON
CALORIES: 19 • CHOL.: 0 • FAT: 1 G. • SODIUM: 11 MG.

Lois's Cranberry Conserve

Just about the most-special cranberry accompaniment ever made.
So good it's sometimes given as a gift for Thanksgiving or Christmas.

Prepare Ahead • Gourmet

    4 cups CRANBERRIES
    I cup WATER
    2-1/2 cups SUGAR
    I cup PECANS**, cut up or broken in half
    I cup whole seedless RAISINS**
    I small ORANGE**, put through grater or blender

Cook cranberries in 1 cup of water until the skins burst, approximately 10 to 15 minutes. Cool, then put through blender and then sieve.

Bring strained cranberries and sugar to a boil, then add pecans, raisins, and orange. Return to a boil, and immediately remove from heat. Let stand until cool.

Prepare a few days before so flavors can blend. Serve cold.

MAKES I QUART TO 5 CUPS
SERVING SIZE: 2 TABLESPOONS
CALORIES: 75 • CHOL.: 0 • FAT: TRACE • SODIUM: 30 MG.

---

*=Dangerous to some • **=Consume with caution • See pages 19-22 for more information

Breads, Muffins, & Breakfasts

Crunchy Bread Sticks

Adding a bread variation to a meal can make it special;
poppy seeds could also be used.

Quick and Easy

Onion powder**

2 Tbsp. MARGARINE
1/2 tsp. DRIED DILL WEED
dash ONION POWDER**
2 slices WHITE BREAD

Preheat oven to 350 degrees. Melt margarine and mix in dill weed and onion powder. Trim crust from bread and brush both sides of slices with margarine mixture. Cut each slice into 4 strips. Set on an ungreased baking sheet and bake for 12 to 15 minutes, turning once, or until golden brown and crisp.

SESAME STICKS: Substitute 2 tablespoons sesame seed for dill weed and onion powder.

MAKES 8 BREAD STICKS
SERVING SIZE: 1 BREAD STICK

CRUNCHY BREAD STICKS
CALORIES: 41 • CHOL.: 0 • FAT: 3 G. • SODIUM: 54 MG.

SESAME STICKS
CALORIES: 54 • CHOL.: 0 • FAT: 4 G. • SODIUM: 54 MG.

Date-and-Nut Bread

With this very special sliced bread in the freezer, you'll always be ready
for drop-in guests. It stays moist and wonderful, frozen, even up to one year!
Makes a special meal or a great small sandwich with cream cheese or margarine.

Prepare Ahead • Gourmet

Vanilla extract*, Walnuts**, Pecans**, Dates*

3/4 cup chopped WALNUTS** or PECANS**

I cup cut up, pitted DATES*

1-1/2 tsp. BAKING SODA

1/2 tsp. SALT

3 Tbsp. SHORTENING

3/4 cup boiling WATER

2 EGGS or 1/2 cup EGG SUBSTITUTE

I tsp. VANILLA*

I cup SUGAR

1-1/2 cups sifted ALL-PURPOSE FLOUR

With fork, mix walnuts, dates, soda, and salt. Add shortening and water;
let stand 20 minutes. Preheat oven to 350 degrees. Grease 9 x 5 x 3-inch
loaf pan. With fork, beat eggs; beat in vanilla, sugar, and flour. Mix in date
mixture until just blended; turn into pan. Bake 1 hour and 5 minutes, or
until wooden toothpick inserted in center comes out clean. Cool in pan
10 minutes; remove. Cool overnight before slicing. Freezes beautifully!

MAKES I LOAF
SERVING SIZE: I SLICE (3/16 INCH)
CALORIES: 124 • CHOL.: 0.2 MG. • FAT: 2.4 G. • SODIUM: 128 MG.

---

*=Dangerous to some • **=Consume with caution • See pages 19-22 for more information

Low-Salt Challah

Try this yeast bread. The less flour used in kneading, the more tender the challah.

Prepare Ahead • Gourmet

I cup WARM WATER (105 to 115 degrees)
I pkg. ACTIVE DRY YEAST
2 Tbsp. SUGAR
dash POWDERED SAFFRON (optional)
1/2 cup SWEET UNSALTED MARGARINE, melted and slightly cooled
3/4 cup EGG SUBSTITUTE (room temperature), or 3 EGGS
5-1/4 to 5-3/4 cups ALL-PURPOSE FLOUR
2 tsp. EGG SUBSTITUTE
POPPY SEED

Measure warm water into large warm bowl. Sprinkle in yeast; stir until dissolved. Stir in sugar, saffron, and margarine. Blend in 3/4 cup egg substitute. Add 3 cups flour; beat until smooth. Stir in enough additional flour to form a stiff dough. Turn out onto a lightly floured board; knead until smooth and elastic, about 8 to 10 minutes. Place in a greased bowl, turning to grease top. Cover, and let rise in warm draft-free place until doubled in size, about 1 hour.

Punch dough down; divide in half. Divide each half into 2 pieces, one about 1/3 of dough and the other about 2/3 of dough. Divide larger piece into 3 equal pieces. Roll each piece into a 12-inch rope. Braid the 3 ropes together; pinch ends to seal. Divide smaller piece into 3 equal pieces. Roll each piece into a 10-inch rope. Braid the ropes together; place on top of large braid. Seal braids together at ends. Repeat with remaining dough to form second loaf. Brush braids with 2 teaspoons egg substitute; sprinkle with poppy seed. Cover, and let rise in warm draft-free place until doubled in size, about 1 hour. Bake at 375 degrees for 20 to 25 minutes or until done. Remove from baking sheets and cool on wire racks.

MAKES 2 LOAVES, 18 SLICES PER LOAF
SERVING SIZE: I SLICE
CALORIES: 97 • CHOL.: 0 • FAT: 3 G. • SODIUM: 8 MG.

*=Dangerous to some • **=Consume with caution • See pages 19-22 for more information

Orange "Chocolate" Chip Bread

The orange juice and peel surprisingly complement the carob chips and vice versa.

Prepare Ahead

Orange juice**, Orange peel**, Buttermilk**

1 cup SKIM MILK
1/4 cup ORANGE JUICE**
1/3 cup SUGAR
1 EGG, slightly beaten
1 Tbsp. grated fresh ORANGE PEEL**
3 cups BUTTERMILK BISCUIT MIX**
1/2 cup CAROB CHIPS (semi-sweet kisses)

Preheat oven to 350 degrees. Grease 9 x 5 x 2-3/4-inch loaf pan. In a medium mixing bowl, combine milk, orange juice, sugar, egg, and orange peel; stir into baking mix. Beat until well combined, about 1 minute. Stir in carob chips; pour into prepared pan. Bake 45 to 50 minutes or until wooden toothpick inserted in center comes out clean. Cool 10 minutes; remove from pan. Cool completely.

MAKES 16 SERVINGS
SERVING SIZE: 1 SLICE (1/2 INCH)
CALORIES: 161 • CHOL.: 0 • FAT: 10 G. • SODIUM: 374 MG.

Pecan Sticky Buns

Always a great favorite as you may have noticed in the shopping malls and at fairs. Of course, if nuts are a trigger agent for headaches for you, skip the pecans.

Prepare Ahead • Gourmet

Pecans**

Dough

3-1/4 to 3-3/4 cups ALL-PURPOSE FLOUR
1/4 cup SUGAR
1 pkg. ACTIVE DRY YEAST
1/2 cup SKIM MILK
1/4 cup WATER
1/3 cup MARGARINE
1/2 cup EGG SUBSTITUTE, or 2 EGGS

Topping and filling

6 Tbsp. MARGARINE
1-1/4 cups firmly packed DARK BROWN SUGAR
1/2 cup LIGHT CORN SYRUP
1/2 cup PECAN** pieces

In large bowl, mix 1 cup flour, sugar, and undissolved yeast. In saucepan, heat milk, water, and 1/3 cup margarine to 120 to 130 degrees. Margarine need not melt. Add to dry ingredients and beat 2 minutes at medium speed with mixer, scraping bowl occasionally. Add egg substitute and 1/2 cup flour. Beat at high speed for 2 minutes. Stir in enough additional flour to make a soft dough.

Knead on lightly floured board 8 to 10 minutes. Place in greased bowl, turning dough to grease top. Cover, and let rise in warm draft-free place until doubled, about 1 hour.

While dough is rising, mix 4 tablespoons margarine with 1 cup brown sugar and corn syrup. Cook and stir until sugar dissolves. Pour into ungreased 13 x 9 x 2-inch baking pan. Sprinkle with pecan pieces.

Punch dough down; divide in half. Roll each half to a 14 x 9-inch rectangle. Melt remaining margarine and brush on dough; sprinkle with remaining brown sugar. Roll up to form 9-inch rolls. Pinch seams. Cut each roll into 9 slices. Arrange in prepared pan. Cover; let rise until doubled, about 45 minutes.

Bake at 375 degrees for 20 to 25 minutes or until done. Cool in pan for 5 minutes, then invert onto wire rack to cool completely.

MAKES 18 BUNS
SERVING SIZE: 1 BUN
CALORIES: 274 • CHOL.: 0 • FAT: 9 G. • SODIUM: 83 MG.

Pumpkin Bread

This moist, easy-to-make bread is a winner. It doesn't dry out or pick up flavors from the freezer. It's also easy to slice and won't crumble.

Prepare Ahead • Gourmet

Nuts**, Raisins*

3-1/2 cups FLOUR

3 cups SUGAR

2 tsp. BAKING SODA

1 tsp. BAKING POWDER

1-1/2 tsp. SALT

1 tsp. CINNAMON

1 tsp. NUTMEG

2/3 cup WATER

1 cup OIL

4 EGGS

2 cups canned PUMPKIN

1 cup chopped NUTS**

1 cup RAISINS*

Preheat oven to 350 degrees. Sift all dry ingredients (including sugar) together into a large mixing bowl. Make a well in the center, and add remaining ingredients except raisins and nuts. Mix thoroughly. Add raisins and nuts; stir well.

Pour mixture into three greased and floured bread loaf pans and bake for 1 hour. Let cool slightly before removing from pans. Slice, wrap in foil, and store in the refrigerator. This bread may be frozen for up to 1 year.

MAKES 3 LOAVES

SERVING SIZE: 1 SLICE (3/16 INCH)

CALORIES: 118 • CHOL.: 0.1 MG. • FAT: 3 G. • SODIUM: 126 MG.

Salt-Free Whole Wheat Bread

Whole wheat flour makes a closer-grained, less fluffy loaf because the whole wheat bran cuts the yeast-rising strands; it has a close, solid structure compared to white bread.

Prepare Ahead

4-1/2 to 5 cups ALL-PURPOSE FLOUR
2 cups WHOLE WHEAT FLOUR
1 Tbsp. SUGAR
2 pkgs. ACTIVE DRY YEAST
2-1/4 cups WATER
1/4 cup HONEY
1/3 cup SWEET UNSALTED MARGARINE

Combine flours. In a large bowl thoroughly mix 2 cups flour mixture, sugar, and undissolved yeast.

In saucepan, heat water, honey, and margarine until very warm (120 to 130 degrees). Margarine does not need to melt. Gradually add to dry ingredients and beat 2 minutes at medium speed with electric mixer, scraping bowl occasionally. Stir in enough additional flour mixture to make a stiff dough. Turn out onto a lightly floured board and knead until smooth and elastic, about 8 to 10 minutes. Place in greased bowl, turning dough to grease top. Cover; let rise in warm draft-free place until doubled in size, about 40 minutes.

Punch dough down; turn out onto a lightly floured board. Divide dough in half. Shape each half into a loaf. Place in 2 greased 8-1/2 x 4-1/2 x 2-1/2-inch or 9 x 5 x 3-inch loaf pans. Cover; let rise in a warm draft-free place until doubled in size, about 45 minutes. Bake at 400 degrees for 30 to 35 minutes or until done. Remove from pans and cool on wire racks.

MAKES 2 LOAVES, 15 SLICES PER LOAF
SERVING SIZE: 1 SLICE
CALORIES: 128 • CHOL.: 0 • FAT: 2 G. • SODIUM: 1 MG.

Soft Poppy Seed Loaf

A delicious bread with its delicate almond, poppy seed, and orange flavors.

Prepare Ahead • Gourmet

**Vanilla and Almond extracts*,
Orange juice**, Orange peel***

1/2 tsp. SALT
3 cups FLOUR
2 tsp. VANILLA EXTRACT*
3/4 cup VEGETABLE OIL
1/2 cup FROZEN ORANGE JUICE CONCENTRATE**, thawed
1-1/2 tsp. BAKING POWDER
1-1/2 cups SUGAR
1-1/2 cups SKIM MILK
1-1/2 tsp. ALMOND EXTRACT*
2 Tbsp. POPPY SEEDS
3/4 cup EGG SUBSTITUTE, or 3 EGGS
1 Tbsp. finely grated ORANGE PEEL**
2 Tbsp. POWDERED SUGAR
NONSTICK COOKING SPRAY

Preheat oven to 350 degrees. Combine all ingredients except orange peel and powdered sugar in a large mixing bowl. Beat for 2 minutes. Spray 2 loaf pans with cooking spray. Divide batter between loaf pans and bake for 55 minutes. Remove from pans. Sprinkle with orange peel and powdered sugar while warm.

MAKES 2 LOAVES (18 SLICES EACH)
SERVING SIZE: 1 SLICE
CALORIES: 125 • CHOL.: 1 MG. • FAT: 5 G. • SODIUM: 31 MG.

Confetti Muffins

A quick bread and easy to make.

Prepare Ahead

Raspberries**, Nuts**, Lemon peel**

Nut Topping

   1/3 cup firmly packed BROWN SUGAR
   1/4 cup chopped NUTS**
   1/4 cup FLOUR
   1 tablespoon LIGHT MARGARINE
   1/2 tsp. CINNAMON

Muffins

   NONSTICK COOKING SPRAY
   1 cup FLOUR
   1/2 cup OAT BRAN
   1/4 cup GRANULATED SUGAR
   1/4 cup firmly packed BROWN SUGAR
   2 tsp. BAKING POWDER
   1 tsp. CINNAMON
   1/4 tsp. SALT
   2 EGG WHITES
   1/2 cup light MARGARINE
   1/2 cup SKIM MILK
   1 cup fresh (or frozen unsweetened) RASPBERRIES**
   1 tsp. grated LEMON PEEL**

In small bowl, combine topping ingredients. Mix with fork until crumbly. Set aside.

Preheat oven to 350 degrees. Spray 12 (2-1/2 inch) muffin cups with cooking spray. In medium bowl combine flour, oat bran, sugars, baking powder, cinnamon, and salt. In large bowl mix egg whites, margarine and milk until blended. Stir in flour mixture just until moistened. Fold in raspberries and lemon peel. (If frozen raspberries are used, they must be thawed and well drained.) Spoon batter into paper-lined muffin cups.
   continued…

---

*=Dangerous to some • **=Consume with caution • See pages 19-22 for more information

Sprinkle each with nut topping. Bake 20 to 25 minutes or until lightly browned and firm to the touch. Cool in pan on wire rack 5 minutes. Remove from pan.

MAKES 12 MUFFINS
SERVING SIZE: 1 MUFFIN
CALORIES: 180 • CHOL.: 0 • FAT: 6 G. • SODIUM: 220 MG.

Applesauce Spice Muffins

Moist, luscious muffins. Be careful not to over-beat the batter as that creates tunnels and a tougher product.

Quick and Easy

Cream Cheese Frosting

1-1/2 oz. (3 Tbsp.) LOW-FAT CREAM CHEESE
1 tsp. MILK
1 cup POWDERED SUGAR

Muffins

NONSTICK COOKING SPRAY
1/2 cup WHOLE WHEAT FLOUR
1/2 cup ALL-PURPOSE FLOUR
1-1/2 tsp. CINNAMON
1 tsp. BAKING SODA
1/4 tsp. GROUND CLOVES
1 cup UNSWEETENED APPLESAUCE
3/4 cup firmly packed BROWN SUGAR
1/3 cup VEGETABLE OIL
1 EGG or 1/4 cup EGG SUBSTITUTE

Preheat oven to 350 degrees. In small bowl with mixer at low speed, beat frosting ingredients until blended. Beat on high speed 1 minute or until smooth. Preheat oven to 350 degrees. Spray 12 (2-1/2 inch) muffin cups with cooking spray. In small bowl combine flours, cinnamon, baking soda and cloves. In medium bowl, mix applesauce, brown sugar, oil and egg until smooth. Pour into flour mixture. Stir just until dry ingredients are dampened. Spoon into paper-lined muffin cups; bake in 350 degree oven 18 minutes or until lightly browned and firm to the touch. Cool in pan on wire rack 5 minutes. Remove from pan, cool completely. Spread with cream cheese frosting.

MAKES 12 MUFFINS
SERVING SIZE: 1 FROSTED MUFFIN
CALORIES: 210 • CHOL.: 20 MG. • FAT: 8 G. • SODIUM: 95 MG.

*=Dangerous to some • **=Consume with caution • See pages 19-22 for more information

Quick "Chocolate" Muffins

*The oil in this recipe helps to make the muffins tender
and free from tunnels and peaking.*

Quick and Easy

Vanilla extract*

1-1/2 cups ALL-PURPOSE FLOUR
1 cup SUGAR
1/4 cup CAROB POWDER
1 tsp. BAKING SODA
1/2 tsp. SALT
1 cup WATER
1/4 cup plus 2 Tbsp. VEGETABLE OIL
1 Tbsp. WHITE VINEGAR
1 tsp. VANILLA EXTRACT*

Preheat oven to 375 degrees. In medium mixing bowl, combine flour, sugar, carob powder, baking soda, and salt. Add water, oil, vinegar, and vanilla. Stir by hand just until dry ingredients are dampened. Pour batter into paper-lined muffin pans (2-1/2 inch in diameter), filling each 2/3 full. Bake 16 to 18 minutes or until wooden toothpick inserted in center comes out clean. Cool in pan for 5 minutes, then remove from pan and cool completely. Frost if desired.

MAKES ABOUT 18 MUFFINS
SERVING SIZE: 1 MUFFIN
CALORIES: 129 • CHOL.: 0 • FAT: 5 G. • SODIUM: 121 MG.

Whole Grain Muffins

These muffins aren't just tasty, they're nutritious, too.
The oats and oat bran are also cholesterol-lowering agents.

Quick and Easy

NONSTICK COOKING SPRAY
1-1/2 cups SKIM MILK
3/4 cup uncooked OAT BRAN CEREAL
1/4 cup EGG SUBSTITUTE, or 1 EGG
BROWN SUGAR SUBSTITUTE equivalent to 1/4 cup brown sugar
1 Tbsp. plus 1 tsp. VEGETABLE OIL
1 cup QUICK-COOKING or REGULAR ROLLED OATS
1 cup WHOLE WHEAT FLOUR
1 Tbsp. BAKING POWDER

Preheat oven to 400 degrees. Spray 12 (2-1/2 inch) muffin cups with cooking spray, or line each with a paper baking cup. In a medium bowl, combine milk and oat bran cereal. Add egg substitute, brown sugar substitute, and oil. Mix well. In a small bowl, combine remaining ingredients. Add to oat bran mixture. Mix until dry ingredients are moistened. Spoon into prepared muffin cups, filling 2/3 full. Bake about 20 minutes or until light brown. Cool in pan for 5 minutes, then remove from pan and cool completely.

MAKES 12 MUFFINS
SERVING SIZE: 1 MUFFIN
CALORIES: 103 • CHOL.: 1 MG. • FAT: 3.3 G. • SODIUM: 132 MG.

French Coffee Cake

Try this coffee cake for an inexpensive late evening snack, breakfast, or guests.

Prepare Ahead • Gourmet

Vanilla extract*, Yogurt**, Nuts**

Coffee Cake

NONSTICK COOKING SPRAY
1 cup DIET MARGARINE
1-1/4 cups SUGAR
2 cups PLAIN NONFAT YOGURT**
3 EGG WHITES
1-1/2 tsp. VANILLA EXTRACT*
3 cups FLOUR
1-1/2 tsp. BAKING POWDER
1 tsp. BAKING SODA

Filling

1/2 cup chopped WALNUTS** or PECANS** (optional)
1/4 cup firmly packed BROWN SUGAR
1/4 cup GRANULATED SUGAR
1-1/2 teaspoons CINNAMON

In small bowl combine filling ingredients. Mix with a fork until crumbly. Set aside.

Preheat oven to 350 degrees. Spray 10-inch Bundt or 10 x 4-inch tube pan with cooking spray. In medium bowl with mixer at medium speed beat margarine and sugar until fluffy. Add yogurt, egg whites, and vanilla; mix thoroughly. Combine flour, baking powder, and baking soda. Gradually add to yogurt mixture, mixing well. Pour 1/3 of the batter into prepared pan. Sprinkle with half the filling. Repeat layers, ending with batter.

Bake in 350 degree oven 65 minutes or until toothpick inserted in center of cake comes out clean. Cool completely in pan on wire rack.

MAKES 24 SERVINGS
SERVING SIZE: 1/4-INCH SLICE
CALORIES: 180 • CHOL.: 0 • FAT: 5 G. • SODIUM: 160 MG.

*=Dangerous to some • **=Consume with caution • See pages 19-22 for more information

French Toast

An old-time favorite with young and old that's nice for breakfast variety.

Quick and Easy

Vanilla extract*

1 cup EGG SUBSTITUTE, or 4 EGGS, beaten
1/3 cup SKIM MILK
1 tsp. GROUND CINNAMON
1 tsp. VANILLA EXTRACT*
2 Tbsp. MARGARINE
10 slices LOW-SODIUM WHITE BREAD
MAPLE FLAVORED SYRUP, optional

In shallow bowl, combine egg substitute, milk, cinnamon, and vanilla. In nonstick skillet over medium heat, melt 2 teaspoons margarine. Dip bread slices in egg substitute mixture to coat; transfer to skillet. Brown about 3 minutes on each side, adding remaining margarine to skillet as needed. Serve with syrup, if desired.

MAKES 5 SERVINGS
SERVING SIZE: 2 SLICES (WITHOUT SYRUP)
CALORIES: 189 • CHOL.: 0 • FAT: 6 G. • SODIUM: 121 MG.

---

*=Dangerous to some • **=Consume with caution • See pages 19-22 for more information

Fruit Blintzes

An ethnic specialty to try for a change from the ordinary.

Specialty

Prunes*

3/4 cup SKIM MILK
I cup ALL-PURPOSE FLOUR
I cup EGG SUBSTITUTE, or 4 EGGS
1/3 cup MARGARINE
I can (16 oz.) sliced PEACHES, well drained and diced
1/2 cup chopped cooked PRUNES*

Alternately add skim milk and flour to egg substitute, mixing until well combined.

Melt 1 teaspoon margarine in a 6-inch skillet. Pour in a thin covering of prepared batter (about 2 tablespoons) just to cover bottom of pan. Tilt pan from side to side to distribute batter evenly. Cook on one side until batter blisters. Turn out onto a clean cloth or waxed paper. Repeat with remaining batter to make 16 blintzes, using melted margarine as needed.

Combine peaches and prunes. Place 1 tablespoonful of mixture on each blintz. Fold in sides to form a square. Melt 2 tablespoons margarine in a large skillet. Brown squares on both sides. Serve hot.

MAKES 16 BLINTZES
SERVING SIZE: I BLINTZ
CALORIES: 91 • CHOL.: 0 • FAT: 4 G. • SODIUM: 59 MG.

Gingerbread Raisin Pancakes

If you like ginger, you'll appreciate these pancakes. Like muffins, over-stirring causes a tougher product. The first pancakes prepared are the most tender.

Quick and Easy

Raisins*

1-1/4 cups FLOUR
1 tsp. BAKING POWDER
1/2 tsp. BAKING SODA
1/2 tsp. SALT
1/2 tsp. CINNAMON
1/4 tsp. GROUND GINGER
1 EGG
1 cup SKIM MILK
1/4 cup MOLASSES
3 Tbsp. MARGARINE, melted
1/3 cup RAISINS*
NONSTICK COOKING SPRAY

In medium bowl combine flour, baking powder, baking soda, salt, cinnamon, and ginger. In small bowl mix egg, milk, molasses, and margarine until blended. Add egg mixture to flour mixture, stirring just until moistened. Stir in raisins.

Spray griddle with cooking spray; heat. For each pancake, pour scant 1/4 cup batter onto hot griddle. Cook over medium heat, turning once, 4 minutes or until browned.

MAKES 4 SERVINGS
SERVING SIZE: 3 (4-INCH) PANCAKES
CALORIES: 350 • CHOL.: 55 MG. • FAT: 10 G. • SODIUM: 590 MG.

Jam Toast Triangles

A juicy, easy-to-make breakfast or supper dish enjoyed by both children and adults.

Quick and Easy

---

10 tsp. PRESERVES or JAM, any flavor except raspberry, orange, or fig
5 slices BREAD
1/4 cup EGG SUBSTITUTE, or 1 EGG
1/4 cup SKIM MILK
2 Tbsp. MARGARINE
1/4 tsp. GROUND CINNAMON
1 Tbsp. SUGAR

Spread 2 teaspoons preserves onto each slice of bread. Cut each slice diagonally in half. Place one half over the other to form a sandwich; press to seal. In medium bowl, combine egg substitute and skim milk. Dip each sandwich in egg mixture to coat. In medium skillet over medium-high heat, melt margarine. Add sandwiches; cook until toasted on both sides.

Combine sugar and cinnamon; sprinkle over sandwiches. Serve warm.

MAKES 5 SERVINGS
SERVING SIZE: 1 SANDWICH
CALORIES: 166 • CHOL.: 1 MG. • FAT: 5 G. • SODIUM: 285 MG.

Vegetable Omelet

A quick-to-prepare omelet with colorful vegetables and no cholesterol.
Use 1/2 cup egg substitute, if preferred.

Quick and Easy

Onion** or Chives**

1 tsp. OLIVE OIL
3 Tbsp. finely diced BROCCOLI
2 Tbsp. finely diced RED or GREEN PEPPER
1 tsp. finely diced ONION** or CHIVES**
1/4 cup EGG SUBSTITUTE
SALT and PEPPER to taste

Combine olive oil, broccoli, pepper, and onion in frying pan. Cook over medium heat for about 2 minutes, stirring constantly. Pour egg substitute over vegetables and cook until thickened but still moist. Serve immediately.

MAKES 1 SERVING
SERVING SIZE: 1 OMELET
CALORIES: 84 • CHOL.: 0 • FAT: 4.6 G. • SODIUM: 115 MG.

*=Dangerous to some • **=Consume with caution • See pages 19-22 for more information

Omelet Primavera

*Omelets seem to make any meal special. They are suitable for
a summer luncheon or evening meal as well as breakfast.*

Quick and Easy

Mushrooms*

2 tsp. MARGARINE
1/2 cup sliced YELLOW SQUASH
1/2 cup sliced ZUCCHINI
1/4 cup RED PEPPER STRIPS
1/4 cup GREEN PEPPER STRIPS
1 cup sliced MUSHROOMS*
1 container (8 oz.) EGG SUBSTITUTE

Melt 1 teaspoon margarine in an 8-inch nonstick omelet pan over
medium heat. Add vegetables; cook and stir until tender-crisp. Remove
from pan; set aside. In same pan, melt remaining margarine; pour in egg
substitute. Cook, lifting edges to allow uncooked portion to flow under-
neath. When almost set, spoon vegetables over half of omelet. With spatula, fold other half over filling; slide onto serving dish. Serve immediately.

MAKES 2 SERVINGS
SERVING SIZE: 1/2 OMELET
CALORIES: 112 • CHOL.: 0 • FAT: 4 G. • SODIUM: 120 MG.

Breakfast Burrito

A south-of-the-border change from the usual breakfast

Quick and Easy

NONSTICK COOKING SPRAY
1/2 cup EGG SUBSTITUTE, or 2 EGGS
1 CORN TORTILLA
2 Tbsp. CHUNKY SALSA (mild, medium, or hot)

Spray nonstick skillet with cooking spray; pour egg substitute in skillet and cook to desired doneness. Microwave corn tortilla for 30 seconds. Fill tortilla with cooked egg substitute. Top with salsa.

MICROWAVE: Pour egg substitute into small microwave-safe bowl. Cook on medium (60-70% power) for 1 minute or desired doneness. Microwave corn tortilla for 30 seconds. Fill tortilla with cooked egg substitute. Top with salsa.

MAKES 1 SERVING
SERVING SIZE: 1 BURRITO
CALORIES: 92 • CHOL.: 0 • FAT: 1 G. • SODIUM: 340 MG.

Egg Salad on Bagels

Skip the top half of the bagel to reduce the calories.

Quick and Easy

Mayonnaise*, Yogurt**

1 tsp. DIJON MUSTARD
1 Tbsp. "light" MAYONNAISE*
1/2 cup PLAIN NONFAT YOGURT**
1/4 cup chopped CELERY
1/4 tsp. DILL WEED
1 hard-cooked EGG YOLK, chopped
4 hard-cooked EGG WHITES, chopped
4 whole BAGELS, sliced horizontally

In medium bowl, combine all ingredients except eggs and bagels. Add egg whites and yolk; fold in gently. Spread 1/3 cup of mixture on each of 4 bagel halves. Top with remaining bagel halves.

MAKES 4 SERVINGS
SERVING SIZE: 1 SALAD BAGEL
CALORIES: 229 • CHOL.: 70 MG. • FAT: 4 G. • SODIUM: 4 MG.

Toasted Egg Salad Sandwiches
An old favorite minus the cholesterol.

Prepare Ahead

Scallions**

2 cartons (8 oz. each) EGG SUBSTITUTE
1/4 cup CREAMY MAYONNAISE (see page XX)
1/4 cup chopped CELERY
1/4 cup chopped RED PEPPER
2 Tbsp. chopped SCALLIONS**
12 slices LOW-SODIUM WHITE BREAD
6 LETTUCE LEAVES

Pour egg substitute into large nonstick skillet. Cover tightly; cook over very low heat 10 minutes or just until set. Remove from heat; let stand, covered, for 10 minutes. Remove from skillet, and cool completely; Coarsely chop.

In bowl, combine hard-cooked egg substitute, mayonnaise, celery, red pepper, and scallions. Cover; chill until serving time. Divide and spread on 6 toasted bread slices; top with lettuce and remaining bread. Serve immediately.

MAKES 6 SERVINGS
SERVING SIZE: 1 SANDWICH
CALORIES: 238 • CHOL. 0 • FAT: 8 G. • SODIUM: 127 MG.

---

*=Dangerous to some • **=Consume with caution • See pages 19-22 for more information

Desserts & Sweets

Baked Apple Crumble

You may have known the old-fashioned favorite as Apple Betty. Instead of baking in an oiled casserole, a pie shell can be substituted if you prefer pastry.

Easy

Orange juice**, Yogurt** (optional)

Apple layer

NONSTICK COOKING SPRAY
6 cups sliced, peeled APPLES (about 2 lbs. or 6 medium apples)
2 Tbsp. ORANGE JUICE** or other fruit juice
3/4 cup firmly packed LIGHT BROWN SUGAR
1/2 cup ALL-PURPOSE FLOUR
1/2 tsp. CINNAMON
3 Tbsp. VEGETABLE OIL

Topping (optional)

1/2 cup LOW-FAT VANILLA YOGURT**, divided

Preheat oven to 375 degrees. Arrange apples evenly in a 2-quart casserole or baking dish coated with cooking spray. Drizzle with orange juice. Combine brown sugar, flour, and cinnamon. Mix in oil until crumbly. Spoon over apples. Bake for 35 minutes or until apples are tender. Cool slightly; serve warm. If desired, spoon one tablespoon vanilla yogurt over each serving.

MAKES 8 SERVINGS
SERVING SIZE: 2/3 CUP
CALORIES: 200 • CHOL.: 0 • FAT: 6 G. • SODIUM: 10 MG.

---

*=Dangerous to some • **=Consume with caution • See pages 19-22 for more information

Banana Cream Pie

Your family or guest may go ape over this pie and only you know that the sugar-free pudding mix, skim milk, and low-calorie topping mix keep the calorie count down.

Prepare Ahead

Vanilla extract*, Bananas**

Crust

> 7 large GRAHAM CRACKERS, crushed
> 3 Tbsp. MARGARINE, melted
> 2 packets SWEETENER

Combine graham cracker crumbs, margarine, and sweetener in a small bowl. Using the back of a spoon, press crumb mixture into a 9-inch pie plate. Chill 3 hours or more.

Filling

> 1 envelope REDUCED-CALORIE WHIPPED TOPPING MIX
> 1 4-serving size box INSTANT SUGAR-FREE VANILLA PUDDING MIX
> 2 cups SKIM MILK
> 1/2 tsp. VANILLA EXTRACT*
> 3 medium BANANAS** (not overly ripe)

Prepare whipped topping mix according to package directions. In a separate bowl, prepare pudding with milk according to package directions. Add vanilla. Fold topping into pudding. Slice bananas and arrange in pie crust. Top with pudding mixture. Chill several hours before serving.

MAKES 10 SERVINGS
SERVING SIZE: 1/10 OF PIE
CALORIES: 165 • CHOL.: 0 • FAT: 6 G. • SODIUM: 276 MG.

---

*=Dangerous to some • **=Consume with caution • See pages 19-22 for more information

Banana Snacking Cake

Note that this moist cake is cholesterol-free. Avoid bananas that are over-ripe; they contain more of the blood pressure agent, tyramine.

Prepare Ahead

Bananas**, Walnuts**, Yogurt**

2-1/4 cups ALL-PURPOSE FLOUR
2 tsp. BAKING POWDER
1 tsp. BAKING SODA
1/3 cup MARGARINE, softened
1-1/4 cups SUGAR
3/4 cup EGG SUBSTITUTE, or 3 EGGS
1-1/4 cups mashed BANANAS** (about 2 large)
2/3 cup PLAIN NONFAT YOGURT**
1/2 cup WALNUTS**, chopped (optional)
CONFECTIONER'S SUGAR (optional)

Preheat oven to 350 degrees. In small bowl, combine flour, baking powder and baking soda; set aside. In large bowl, with electric mixer at medium speed, beat margarine and white sugar until well combined. At low speed, blend in egg substitute and bananas. Add flour mixture alternately with yogurt, mixing until smooth. Stir in walnuts, if desired.

Spoon batter into greased and floured 13 x 9 x 2-inch baking pan. Bake for 45 minutes, or until toothpick inserted in center comes out clean. Cool in pan on wire rack. Dust with confectioner's sugar, if desired, before serving.

MAKES 24 SERVINGS
SERVING SIZE: 2 X 2 INCH SQUARE
CALORIES: 129 • CHOL.: 0 • FAT: 3 G. • SODIUM: 98 MG.

Brown Edge Wafers

These are similar to the vanilla wafers so popular on supermarket shelves. They also taste like un-iced Christmas cookies.

Quick and Easy

Vanilla extract*, Lemon rind**

1/2 cup MARGARINE
1/2 cup SUGAR
3 Tbsp. EGG SUBSTITUTE, or 1 EGG
1 tsp. VANILLA EXTRACT*
1/4 tsp. grated LEMON RIND**
1 cup ALL-PURPOSE FLOUR

Preheat oven to 375 degrees. In small bowl of electric mixer, cream margarine and sugar until light and fluffy. Beat in egg substitute, vanilla, and lemon rind until smooth. Gradually add flour, beating until well blended.

Drop dough by teaspoonsful onto greased baking sheets; flatten slightly. Bake for 7 minutes or until done. Carefully remove from baking sheets and cool on wire racks.

MAKES 4 DOZEN
SERVING SIZE: 2 WAFERS
CALORIES: 35 • CHOL.: 0 • FAT: 2 G. • SODIUM: 18 MG.

Cannoli Cream

This creamy yet crunchy dessert supplies good nutrition in that important mineral, calcium. Be sure the raisins are fresh—less likely to instigate a headache!

Easy • Prepare Ahead

Raisins*, Rum extract**, Orange marmalade**

1 lb. PART-SKIM RICOTTA or COTTAGE CHEESE
1/4 cup SKIM MILK
1/4 cup ORANGE MARMALADE**
1/2 tsp. RUM EXTRACT**
1/3 cup soft GOLDEN RAISINS*
1/4 cup slivered MACADAMIA NUTS

In a blender or food processor, blend ricotta cheese, milk, marmalade, and rum flavoring until smooth. Stir in raisins. Refrigerate 1 hour or longer. Stir in macadamia nuts before serving. Divide mixture among 8 stemmed glasses.

MAKES 8 SERVINGS
SERVING SIZE: 3/4 CUP
CALORIES: 159 • CHOL.: 3 MG. • FAT: 7 G. • SODIUM: 83 MG.

---

*=Dangerous to some • **=Consume with caution • See pages 19-22 for more information

Caramel Custard with Egg Substitute

This popular custard, served around the world, can be served in the custard cups without inverting over individual plates, if you prefer.

Prepare Ahead

Vanilla extract*

6 Tbsp. SUGAR
2-2/3 cups SKIM MILK, scalded
3/4 cup EGG SUBSTITUTE, or 3 EGGS, beaten
1/3 cup SUGAR
3/4 tsp. VANILLA EXTRACT*

Preheat oven to 350 degrees. Melt 6 tablespoons sugar in a small skillet over low to medium heat until golden brown; pour at once into 6 (6 oz.) heatproof custard cups. Tilt dishes to coat evenly; set aside.

Scald milk (heat milk in saucepan over low heat until bubbles form around the edges). Combine egg substitute and 1/3 cup sugar; stir in scalded milk and vanilla. Slowly pour into custard cups. Set cups in a shallow baking pan filled 1-inch deep with hot water. Bake for 25 to 30 minutes or until a knife inserted in center comes out clean; cool to room temperature. Chill 2 hours or until firm.

To serve, loosen edges with a knife and invert over individual plates.

MAKES 6 SERVINGS
SERVING SIZE: 1/2 CUP
CALORIES: 139 • CHOL.: 2 MG. • FAT: 1 G. • SODIUM: 107 MG.

Carrot Cake

A lower-calorie, moist, easy-to-prepare favorite.

Prepare Ahead

Raisins*, Coconut and Vanilla extracts*

Cake

2/3 cup SWEETENER
1/2 cup VEGETABLE OIL
2 EGGS
1 cup FLOUR
1 tsp. BAKING SODA
1/2 tsp. CINNAMON
1/2 tsp. SALT
1 cup grated CARROTS
1/2 cup chopped MACADAMIA NUTS
1/2 cup RAISINS* (fresh, not aged)

Preheat oven to 350 degrees. Grease 8 x 8-inch glass pan. Combine sweetener, vegetable oil, and eggs in a bowl and beat until blended. Add flour, baking soda, cinnamon, salt, grated carrots, chopped nuts, and raisins. Stir well. Pour mixture in pan. Bake for 35 to 40 minutes. Allow to cool completely before frosting.

Frosting

6 oz. CREAM CHEESE
1/2 tsp. COCONUT EXTRACT*
3 packets SWEETENER
1/2 tsp. VANILLA EXTRACT*

Combine ingredients in a bowl and blend well.

MAKES 16 SERVINGS
SERVING SIZE: 2 X 2 INCH SQUARE
CALORIES: 138 • CHOL.: 34 MG. • FAT: 10 G. • SODIUM: 157 MG.

---

*=Dangerous to some • **=Consume with caution • See pages 19-22 for more information

Cashew Raisin Nuggets

These cookies are tasty and never seem to dry out, even when frozen for two weeks!

Prepare Ahead

Raisins*, Vanilla extract*, Cashews**

1-1/2 cups WHOLE WHEAT FLOUR
1/4 tsp. GROUND CINNAMON
1/2 cup MARGARINE
1/2 cup SUGAR
3 Tbsp. EGG SUBSTITUTE, or 1 EGG
1 tsp. VANILLA EXTRACT*
1/4 cup SKIM MILK
1/2 cup chopped, dry roasted, unsalted CASHEWS**
1/2 cup DARK SEEDLESS RAISINS*

Preheat oven to 375 degrees. Combine flour and cinnamon; set aside. Cream together margarine and sugar on medium speed of electric mixer. Beat in egg substitute and vanilla until light and creamy. Blend flour mixture and skim milk alternately into creamed mixture until smooth. Stir in cashews and raisins.

Drop mixture by rounded teaspoonsful onto ungreased baking sheets. Bake for 10 minutes or until done. Remove cookies from sheets and cool on wire racks.

MAKES 3 DOZEN COOKIES
SERVING SIZE: 1 COOKIE
CALORIES: 68 • CHOL.: 0 • FAT: 3 G. • SODIUM: 25 MG.

"Chocolate" Pudding Parfaits

A very pretty dessert that can be made ahead
of time to top off any luncheon or dinner.

Prepare Ahead

Vanilla extract*, Orange slices**, Orange peel**

2/3 cup SUGAR
1/4 cup CAROB POWDER
3 Tbsp. CORNSTARCH
dash SALT
2 cups SKIM MILK
1 Tbsp. MARGARINE
1 tsp. VANILLA EXTRACT*
1 envelope (1.4 oz.) WHIPPED TOPPING MIX
1/2 cup cold SKIM MILK
1/4 tsp. VANILLA EXTRACT*
1/4 tsp. grated ORANGE PEEL**
ORANGE SLICES** (optional)

In medium saucepan combine sugar, carob powder, cornstarch, and salt; gradually stir in 2 cups skim milk. Cook over medium heat, stirring constantly, until mixture boils; boil and stir 1 minute. Remove from heat; blend in margarine and 1 teaspoon vanilla. Pour into medium bowl. Press plastic wrap onto surface of pudding; chill.

In small bowl combine topping mix, 1/2 cup cold skim milk, and 1/4 teaspoon vanilla; prepare according to package directions. Fold 1/2 cup whipped topping into pudding. Blend orange peel into remaining whipped topping.

Alternately spoon "chocolate" pudding and orange flavored whipped topping into parfait glasses. Chill. Garnish with orange slices, if desired.

MAKES 8 SERVINGS
SERVING SIZE: 2/3 CUP
CALORIES: 176 • CHOL.: 2 MG. • FAT: 4 G. • SODIUM: 93 MG.

*=Dangerous to some • **=Consume with caution • See pages 19-22 for more information

Elegant "Chocolate" Angel Torte

Make this "heavenly" dessert ahead of time. Some markets carry carob powder, but almost all health stores have it on their shelves.

Prepare Ahead

Vanilla extract*

1/3 cup CAROB POWDER
1 pkg. (14.5 oz.) ANGEL FOOD CAKE MIX
1 container (8 oz.) FROZEN FAT-FREE WHIPPED TOPPING MIX
1 tsp. VANILLA EXTRACT*
1 cup STRAWBERRY PURÉE
8 STRAWBERRIES, halved

Combine carob powder and cake mix. Proceed with mixing cake as directed on package. Bake and cool as directed. Slice cooled cake crosswise (horizontally) into four 1-inch slices.

Blend whipped topping with vanilla and strawberry purée. Place bottom cake slice on serving plate; spread with 1/4 of topping. Stack next cake layer; spread with topping. Continue layering cake and topping. Garnish with strawberries. Refrigerate for 1 to 2 hours.

To serve, use sharp serrated knife and cut vertically with a gentle sawing motion.

MAKES 16 SERVINGS
SERVING SIZE: 1/16 OF CAKE
CALORIES: 159 • CHOL.: 0 • FAT: 2 G. • SODIUM: 73 MG.

Fudgy Brownies

In this recipe the margarine may be melted in a heavy saucepan and when just warm, add all the other ingredients. It's quick and easy and a very special treat.

Quick and Easy • Prepare Ahead

Vanilla extract*, Walnuts**

1/4 cup MARGARINE
1/2 cup firmly packed LIGHT BROWN SUGAR
1/2 cup SUGAR
1/2 cup ALL-PURPOSE FLOUR
2 Tbsp. CAROB POWDER
3 Tbsp. EGG SUBSTITUTE, or 1 EGG
1 tsp. VANILLA EXTRACT*
1/4 cup WALNUTS**, chopped

Preheat oven to 350 degrees. Melt margarine. In a large bowl or heavy saucepan combine margarine, sugars, flour, carob powder, and egg substitute until well blended. Stir in vanilla extract and walnuts. Spread batter evenly in a well-greased 8 x 8 x 2-inch baking pan.

Bake for 30 minutes or less. Do not overbake. Brownies will be slightly moist in center and will cling slightly to a wooden toothpick when they are done. Cool in pan on wire rack. Cut into 2-inch squares while warm.

MAKES 16 SERVINGS
SERVING SIZE: 2 X 2 INCH SQUARE
CALORIES: 105 • CHOL.: 0 • FAT: 4 G. • SODIUM: 31 MG.

Glazed Apple Tart

The glaze on the apple tart gives a professional appearance.

Prepare Ahead

Orange marmalade**

SINGLE CRUST FLAKY PASTRY (see page 251)
6 Tbsp. SUGAR
1 Tbsp. CORNSTARCH
1/4 tsp. GROUND CINNAMON
6 cups (about 3 large) thickly sliced, pared baking APPLES
1 Tbsp. MARGARINE
1/2 cup ORANGE MARMALADE**

Preheat oven to 400 degrees. Roll out pastry to a 12-inch circle. Fit into a 9-inch springform pan or pie plate, making edges 3/4-inch high.

Mix sugar, cornstarch, cinnamon, and apple slices. Overlap apple slices in a circular pattern in prepared pastry. Dot with margarine. Cover with foil. Bake for 45 minutes.

Heat marmalade over low heat just until thin. Uncover tart and drizzle over apples. Continue baking tart, uncovered, 15 minutes longer or until apples are tender. Cool.

MAKES 10 SERVINGS
SERVING SIZE: 1/10 OF TART
CALORIES: 230 • CHOL.: 0 • FAT: 7 G. • SODIUM: 62 MG.

Honey Walnut Cake (Lekach)

These bars freeze well and will satisfy anyone's sweet tooth.

Prepare Ahead

Coffee powder*, Walnuts**

1/2 cup MARGARINE
1/2 cup firmly packed LIGHT BROWN SUGAR
1/2 cup HONEY
1/4 cup EGG SUBSTITUTE, or 1 EGG
1 cup ALL-PURPOSE FLOUR
1 tsp. INSTANT COFFEE POWDER*
1/4 tsp. BAKING SODA
1/4 tsp. GROUND CINNAMON
1/4 tsp. GROUND CLOVES
1/4 tsp. GROUND ALLSPICE
1/4 cup SKIM MILK
1/4 cup WALNUTS**, chopped

Preheat oven to 375 degrees. Cream together margarine, brown sugar, and honey. Add egg substitute and continue beating until mixture is fluffy. Mix in flour, instant coffee, baking soda, cinnamon, cloves, allspice, skim milk, and walnuts until well blended.

Spread batter in a greased 8-inch square baking pan. Bake for 30 minutes or until done. Cool in pan on wire rack. Cut into 9 pieces.

MAKES 9 SERVINGS
SERVING SIZE: 2-1/2 INCH SQUARE
CALORIES: 270 • CHOL.: 0 • FAT: 12 G. • SODIUM: 125 MG.

*=Dangerous to some • **=Consume with caution • See pages 19-22 for more information

Lemon Love Notes

A wonderfully tart and delicious treat. An old-fashioned favorite handed down through generations.

Prepare Ahead • Gourmet

Vanilla extract*, Lemon juice**, Lemon rind**

Crust

    1/2 cup MARGARINE
    1/4 cup POWDERED SUGAR
    I cup FLOUR

Preheat oven to 350 degrees. Mix above ingredients well with pastry blender or fork. Put into well-greased 8-inch square pan, lined with greased brown paper. Bake 15 minutes.

Filling

    2 Tbsp. LEMON JUICE**
    1/2 cup EGG SUBSTITUTE, or 2 EGGS, beaten well
    1/2 tsp. BAKING POWDER
    1/2 cup SUGAR
    2 Tbsp. FLOUR
    Grated rind of I LEMON**

Mix above ingredients well and beat. Place on just baked crust; return to 350 degree oven and bake 25 minutes. Cool and frost with:

Thin Icing

    3/4 cup POWDERED SUGAR
    1/2 tsp. VANILLA EXTRACT*
    I Tbsp. MARGARINE
    2 tsp. MILK

Mix thoroughly, and spread over bars.

MAKES 20 SERVINGS
SERVING SIZE: 1-1/2 X 2 INCH BAR
CALORIES: 73 • CHOL.: 0 • FAT: 3 G. • SODIUM: 33 MG.

---

*=Dangerous to some • **=Consume with caution • See pages 19-22 for more information

Mock Rice Pudding

This recipe, with three fruit ingredients, can nutritionally "sweeten" your everyday menu.

Quick and Easy • Prepare Ahead

Mandarin oranges**, Peach yogurt**

I can (10-11 oz.) MANDARIN ORANGES**, drained
I can (10-12 oz.) crushed PINEAPPLE, drained
I APPLE, cored and diced
2 cups cooked WHITE RICE
I carton (8 oz.) LOW-FAT PEACH YOGURT**

Combine all ingredients in bowl; mix. Refrigerate until serving time.

MAKES 6 SERVINGS
SERVING SIZE: 3/4 CUP
CALORIES: 184 • CHOL.: 2 MG. • FAT: I G. • SODIUM: 60 MG.

Saucepan Butterscotch Brownies

A rich, satisfying "brownie" that truly fulfills that sweet-tooth longing.
Admittedly an indulgence for special occasions.

Prepare Ahead

Vanilla extract*, Nuts**

1 stick (or 1/2 cup) MARGARINE
1-1/2 cups BROWN SUGAR, packed
2 EGGS or 1/2 cup EGG SUBSTITUTE
1 tsp. VANILLA EXTRACT*
1-1/2 cups sifted FLOUR
2 tsp. BAKING POWDER
1 cup chopped NUTS**

Preheat oven to 350 degrees. Grease 9 x 13-inch pan. Melt margarine in
a saucepan. Remove from heat. Add brown sugar and blend. Add eggs,
beating well. Stir in vanilla, flour and baking powder. Pour into prepared
pan. Bake about 30 minutes. Do not overbake. Cool in pan and then cut
into bars.

MAKES 24 SERVINGS
SERVING SIZE: 1 1-1/2 X 3 INCH BAR
CALORIES: 115 • CHOL.: 0 • FAT: 5 G. • SODIUM: 98 MG.

---

*=Dangerous to some • **=Consume with caution • See pages 19-22 for more information

Savannah Peach Melba

This dessert can be made ahead of time. Guests will ask for the recipe.

Prepare Ahead

Vanilla extract*, Raspberries**

1 pkg. (3-3/8 oz.) INSTANT VANILLA PUDDING & PIE FILLING, or 1 pkg. (1.7 oz.) SUGAR-FREE INSTANT VANILLA PUDDING & PIE FILLING*

2 cups cold SKIM MILK

1 can (8 oz.) PEACHES, drained and chopped

1 cup fresh or frozen RASPBERRIES**, puréed

2 Tbsp. prepared WHIPPED TOPPING, for garnish

RASPBERRIES** and MINT LEAVES, for garnish

In medium bowl, prepare pudding according to package directions, using skim milk. Stir in peaches. In 4 glasses (8 oz. each) layer pudding mixture and raspberry purée. Chill at least 1 hour. To serve, garnish with whipped topping, raspberries, and mint, if desired.

MAKES 4 SERVINGS

SERVING SIZE: 5 OUNCES

CALORIES: 267 • CHOL.: 10 MG. • FAT: 3 G. • SODIUM: 246 MG.

Single Crust Flaky Pastry

No salt is provided in this recipe (for those on low-sodium diets),
so add 1/8 teaspoon salt to the flour if desired.

Quick and Easy • Prepare Ahead

1/3 cup MARGARINE
1-1/4 cups ALL-PURPOSE FLOUR
3-4 Tbsp. ICE WATER

Cut margarine into flour with pastry cutter or 2 forks until mixture resembles coarse meal. Add 3 to 4 tablespoons ice water, a tablespoon at a time, tossing until moistened. Shape into a ball. Pastry can be chilled until ready to use. Place dough between 2 pieces waxed paper. Roll to fit a 9-inch pie pan, leaving a 1/2-inch crust beyond the edge of the pan.

For recipes requiring a prebaked pie shell, prick pie crust every 2 to 3 inches with a fork to prevent it from blistering. Bake in a 450 degree oven for 12 to 15 minutes or until lightly browned.

MAKES ONE 9-INCH CRUST
NUTRITIONAL VALUE INCLUDED IN RECIPES USING THIS PIE CRUST

Smorgasbord Cheesecake

This truly delicious cheesecake is not exactly inexpensive, but is well worth the cost.

Prepare Ahead • Gourmet

Vanilla extract*, Sour cream**

1/2 lb. CREAM CHEESE
1/3 cup SUGAR
1/2 tsp. VANILLA EXTRACT*
1/2 cup EGG SUBSTITUTE, or 2 EGGS
Few grains SALT

Preheat oven to 275 degrees. Beat the above ingredients together well, then pour into a loaf pan or an 8-inch pie pan. Bake 35 minutes.

Top with a mixture of:
1/2 pint SOUR CREAM**
2-1/2 Tbsp. SUGAR
1/2 tsp. VANILLA EXTRACT*
Few grains SALT

Bake 7 minutes at 275 degrees. Refrigerate.

MAKES 8 SERVINGS (I LOAF PAN)
SERVING SIZE: 1/8 CAKE
CALORIES: 257 • CHOL.: 31 MG. • FAT: 16 G. • SODIUM: 189 MG.

---

*=Dangerous to some • **=Consume with caution • See pages 19-22 for more information

Index

Sources

Alishire, Peter. "Fish Oil or Snake Oil?" Phoenix, Arizona: *The Arizona Republic*, July 22, 1990.

Allen, Ann Moore. *Powers and Moore's Food-Medication Interactions*, Tempe, Arizona: Ann Moore Allen, Publisher, 1991.

Arizona Dietetic Association, Inc. *Arizona Diet Manual*. Phoenix, Arizona: Arizona Department of Health Services, Office of Nutrition Services, and Tucson, Arizona: University of Arizona, College of Medicine, Department of Family and Community Medicine, Health Services Section, 1992.

Blake, Joan Salge. "Can Migraines be Managed Through Diet? Food That May be to Blame." *Environmental Nutrition*, 11:1, 1988.

Brackenridge, Betty Page, R.D. "How to Create a Super Supermarket Shopping Plan." *Diabetes in the News*, 9:3, 1990.

Brainard, John B. *Control of Migraine*, New York: W. W. Norton and Co., 1979.

Diamond, Seymour. "Headaches Can Be a Pain, But Can Be Prevented or Treated." *Diabetes in the News*, 9:3, 1990.

Diet for a Healthy Heart. East Hanover, NJ: Nabisco Brands, Inc., 1988.

Eat Healthy America. Coventry, CT: Best Foods, CPC International, Inc., 1990.

"Food Allergy Network," Phoenix: *The Arizona Republic*, November, 1996.

Goodhart, Robert S. and Shils, Maurice E. *Modern Nutrition in Health and Disease*. New York: Lea and Febiger, 1980.

Grasso, Patricia Holter and Stump, Jan Schaller. *The Headache Cookbook: Tools For Migraine Self-Help*. Bowie, MD: Robert J. Brady Company, 1984.

Griffith, H. Winter. *Complete Guide to Prescription and Non-Prescription Drugs*. Tucson: HP Books, Inc., 1986.

Hanington, E. "Preliminary Report on Tyramine Headaches." *British Medical Journal* 2:550, 1967.

"Healthwatch: Aspirin Regimen May Offer Migraine Relief." Washington, D.C: *A.A.R.P. Bulletin*, 31:6.

Koehler, S. M. and Glaros, A. "The Effect of Aspartame on Migraine Headaches." *Headache*, 28:10, 1988.

Krause, Marie V. and Mahan, L. Kathleen. *Food Nutrition and Diet Therapy*. Philadelphia: W. B. Saunders Company,1984.

McCarthy, Pam, R.D. *Fleishmann's Cholesterol Management Program*, University of Minnesota School of Public Health, 1989.

National Research Council. *Diet and Health Implications for Reducing Chronic Disease Risk*. Washington, D.C: National Academy Press, 1989.

New Light-Style Cooking. Westbury, NY: Pam, 1988.

"New Migraine Research," Phoenix: *The Arizona Republic*, December 26, 1994.

"Nutrition in the Nineties—a Glance Back and a Glimpse Ahead." *On Your Mark*. Washington, D.C: The Sugar Association, Inc., March 1990.

Pappas, Nancy. "Dangerous liaisons: When Food and Drugs Don't Mix." *In Health*, July/August 1990

Pennington, A. T. and Church, Helen Nicholas. *Food Values of Portions Commonly Used*. New York: Harper and Row, Publishers, 1985.

Plenge, Kathern, M.D. *An Ounce of Prevention*. Barrows Neurological Institute, St. Joseph's Hospital and Medical Center, Phoenix, Arizona. VI:3, 1991.

Powers, Dorothy E. and Moore, Ann O. "Food and Medication Interactions." *Food Medication Interactions*, 1988.

"The Sodium Content of Your Food." *Home and Garden Bulletin* Number 233. Washington, D.C: U.S. Government Printing Office, 1982.

Solomon, Neil. Phoenix: Phoenix Newspapers, Inc. March 15, August 25, September 1, 1990.

Stern, Loraine. "Sudden Pain—What Causes It, How to Relieve It; How to Prevent It; When to See a Doctor." *Woman's Day Medical Facts Guide*, Deamandis Communications, Inc., 1989.

Taber, Clarence Wilbur. *Taber's Cyclopedic Medical Dictionary* Philadelphia: F.A. Davis Company, 1985.

Webster, Guy. "Pain Pills May Add to Headache." Phoenix: Phoenix Newspapers, Inc., October 2, 1989.

Wedman, Betty. *Diet and Meal Plans to Control Migraine Headaches*. Fort Atkinson, WI: Nos Co, 1985.

About the Authors

Agnes Peg Hartnell, EdD, RD, is currently a dietetic consultant in private practice. She is the author of four published textbooks about nutrition.

Chairperson emerita of home economics at Phoenix College, Dr. Hartnell has had 25 years experience in teaching, television education, and consultation. Her biography is listed in detail in the 1997-98 edition of *Marquis Who's Who in the West*.

G. Scott Tyler, MD, is a graduate of George Washington University Medical School and was licensed in Colorado and Arizona. In addition to having conducted research for Merck & Company, Sandoz Pharmaceutical Inc. and other companies, he is the former director of the Headache Pain Clinic in Scottsdale, Arizona.

Dr. Tyler has had articles published in significant medical publications, including *Headache*, *Journal of Prosthetic Dentistry*, and *Journal of the Arizona Medical Association*.